Nurse's Medication Notebook

Featuring Twenty-Four Hours

With

Fifteen Minute Increments

Christine Dunne

Christine Dunne, Publisher

Salinas, California 2020

ISBN-978-1-7350162-2-1

Printed by Lulu Press, Inc. in the United States of America

First Printing, 2020

Christine Dunne, Publisher

P.O. Box 2002

Salinas, California 93902

www.deadland.co

Date_____ Patient ID_____ Room Number_____

Medications   Administering   Mathematical

                 Instructions   Computations

EST	Military	Notes	EST	Military	Notes	EST	Military	Notes	EST	Military	Notes
8:00 AM	08:00		3:15PM	15:15		10:15PM	22:15		5:15AM	05:15	
8:15 AM	08:15		3:30PM	15:30		10:30PM	22:30		5:30AM	05:30	
8:30AM	08:30		3:45PM	15:45		10:45PM	22:45		5:45AM	05:45	
8:45AM	08:45		4:00PM	16:00		11:00PM	23:00		6:00AM	06:00	
9:00AM	09:00		4:15PM	16:15		11:15PM	23:15		6:15AM	06:15	
9:15AM	09:15		4:30PM	16:30		11:30PM	23:30		6:30AM	06:30	
9:30AM	09:30		4:45PM	16:45		11:45PM	23:45		6:45AM	06:45	
9:45AM	09:45		5:00PM	17:00		12:00AM	24:00		7:00AM	07:00	
10:00AM	10:00		5:15PM	17:15		12:15AM	24:15		7:15AM	07:15	
10:15AM	10:15		5:30PM	17:30		12:30AM	24:30		730AM	07:30	
10:30AM	10:30		5:45PM	17:45		12:45AM	24:45		7:45AM	07:45	
10:45AM	10:45		6:00PM	18:00		1:00AM	01:00				
11:00AM	11:00		6:15PM	18:15		1:15AM	01:15				
11:15AM	11:15		6:30PM	18:30		1:30AM	01:30				
11:30AM	11:30		6:45PM	18:45		1:45AM	01:45				
11:45AM	11:45		7:00PM	19:00		2:00AM	02:00				
12:00PM	12:00		7:15PM	19:15		2:15AM	02:15				
12:15PM	12:15		7:30PM	19:30		2:45AM	02:45				
12:30PM	12:30		7:45PM	19:45		3:00AM	03:00				
12:45PM	12:45		8:00PM	20:00		3:15AM	03:15				
1:00PM	13:00		8:15PM	20:15		3:30AM	03:30				
1:15PM	13:15		8:30PM	20:30		3:45AM	03:45				
1:30PM	13:30		8:45PM	20:45		4:00AM	04:00				
1:45PM	13:45		9:00PM	21:00		4:15AM	04:15				
2:00PM	14:00		9:15PM	21:15		4:30AM	04:30				
2:15PM	14:15		9:30PM	21:30		4:45AM	04:45				
2:30PM	14:30		9:45PM	21:45		5:00AM	05:00				
2:45PM	14:45		10:00PM	22:00							
3:00PM	15:00										

Date_____ Patient ID_____ Room Number_____

AM MEDS GIVEN? Yes_____

No_____

PM MEDS GIVEN? Yes_____

No_____

Results/Progress Notes:

_____

_____

_____

_____

_____

_____

_____

_____

_____

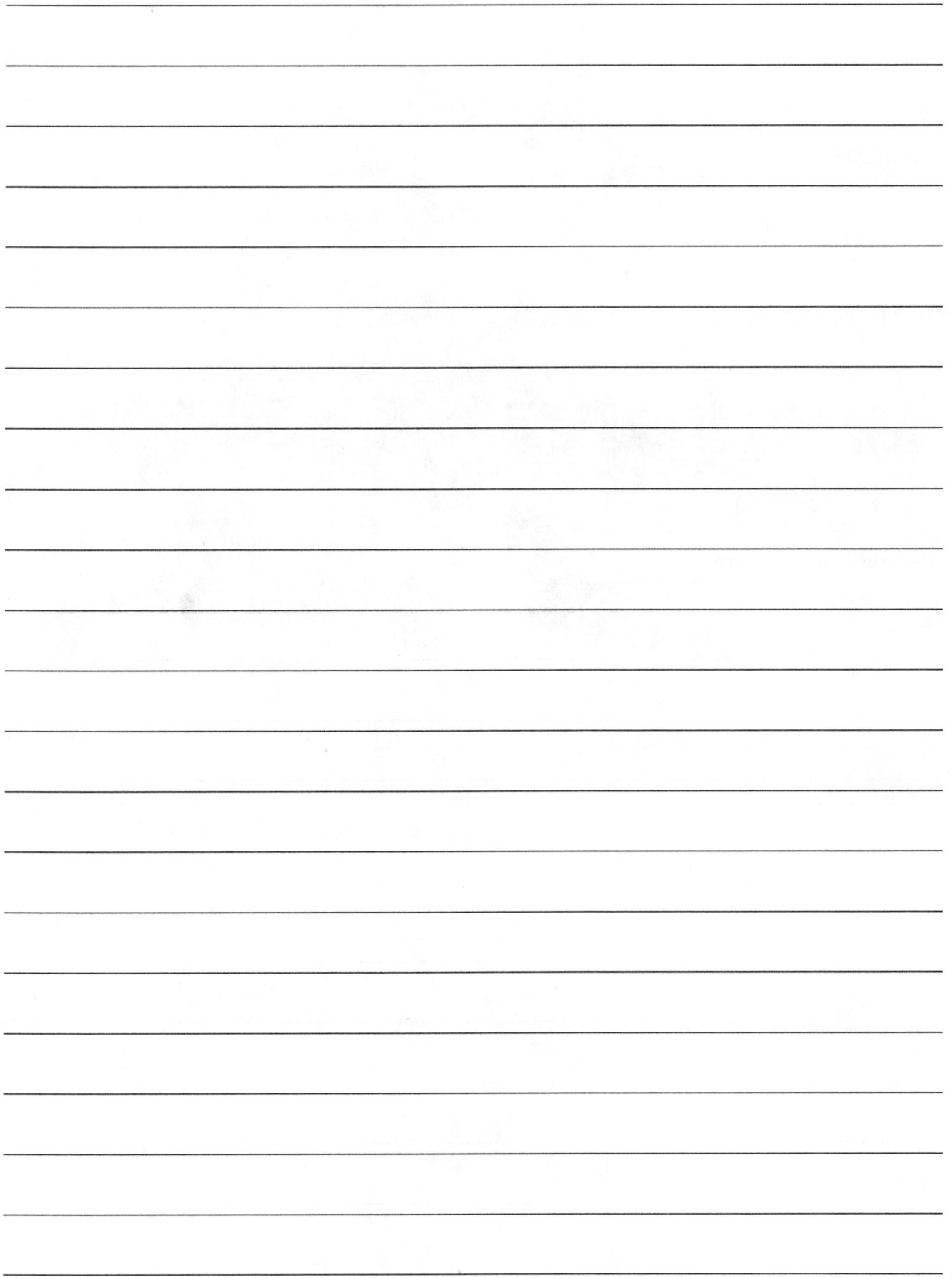

Date_____   Patient ID_____   Room Number_____

Medications	Administering Instructions

Mathematical Computations

EST	Military	Notes	EST	Military	Notes	EST	Military	Notes	EST	Military	Notes
8:00 AM	08:00		3:15PM	15:15		10:15PM	22:15		5:15AM	05:15	
8:15 AM	08:15		3:30PM	15:30		10:30PM	22:30		5:30AM	05:30	
8:30AM	08:30		3:45PM	15:45		10:45PM	22:45		5:45AM	05:45	
8:45AM	08:45		4:00PM	16:00		11:00PM	23:00		6:00AM	06:00	
9:00AM	09:00		4:15PM	16:15		11:15PM	23:15		6:15AM	06:15	
9:15AM	09:15		4:30PM	16:30		11:30PM	23:30		6:30AM	06:30	
9:30AM	09:30		4:45PM	16:45		11:45PM	23:45		6:45AM	06:45	
9:45AM	09:45		5:00PM	17:00		12:00AM	24:00		7:00AM	07:00	
10:00AM	10:00		5:15PM	17:15		12:15AM	24:15		7:15AM	07:15	
10:15AM	10:15		5:30PM	17:30		12:30AM	24:30		730AM	07:30	
10:30AM	10:30		5:45PM	17:45		12:45AM	24:45		7:45AM	07:45	
10:45AM	10:45		6:00PM	18:00		1:00AM	01:00				
11:00AM	11:00		6:15PM	18:15		1:15AM	01:15				
11:15AM	11:15		6:30PM	18:30		1:30AM	01:30				
11:30AM	11:30		6:45PM	18:45		1:45AM	01:45				
11:45AM	11:45		7:00PM	19:00		2:00AM	02:00				
12:00PM	12:00		7:15PM	19:15		2:15AM	02:15				
12:15PM	12:15		7:30PM	19:30		2:45AM	02:45				
12:30PM	12:30		7:45PM	19:45		3:00AM	03:00				
12:45PM	12:45		8:00PM	20:00		3:15AM	03:15				
1:00PM	13:00		8:15PM	20:15		3:30AM	03:30				
1:15PM	13:15		8:30PM	20:30		3:45AM	03:45				
1:30PM	13:30		8:45PM	20:45		4:00AM	04:00				
1:45PM	13:45		9:00PM	21:00		4:15AM	04:15				
2:00PM	14:00		9:15PM	21:15		4:30AM	04:30				
2:15PM	14:15		9:30PM	21:30		4:45AM	04:45				
2:30PM	14:30		9:45PM	21:45		5:00AM	05:00				
2:45PM	14:45		10:00PM	22:00							
3:00PM	15:00										

Date_____   Patient ID_____   Room Number_____

AM MEDS GIVEN? Yes_____

                No_____

PM MEDS GIVEN? Yes_____

                No_____

Results/Progress Notes:

_____

_____

_____

_____

_____

_____

_____

_____

_____

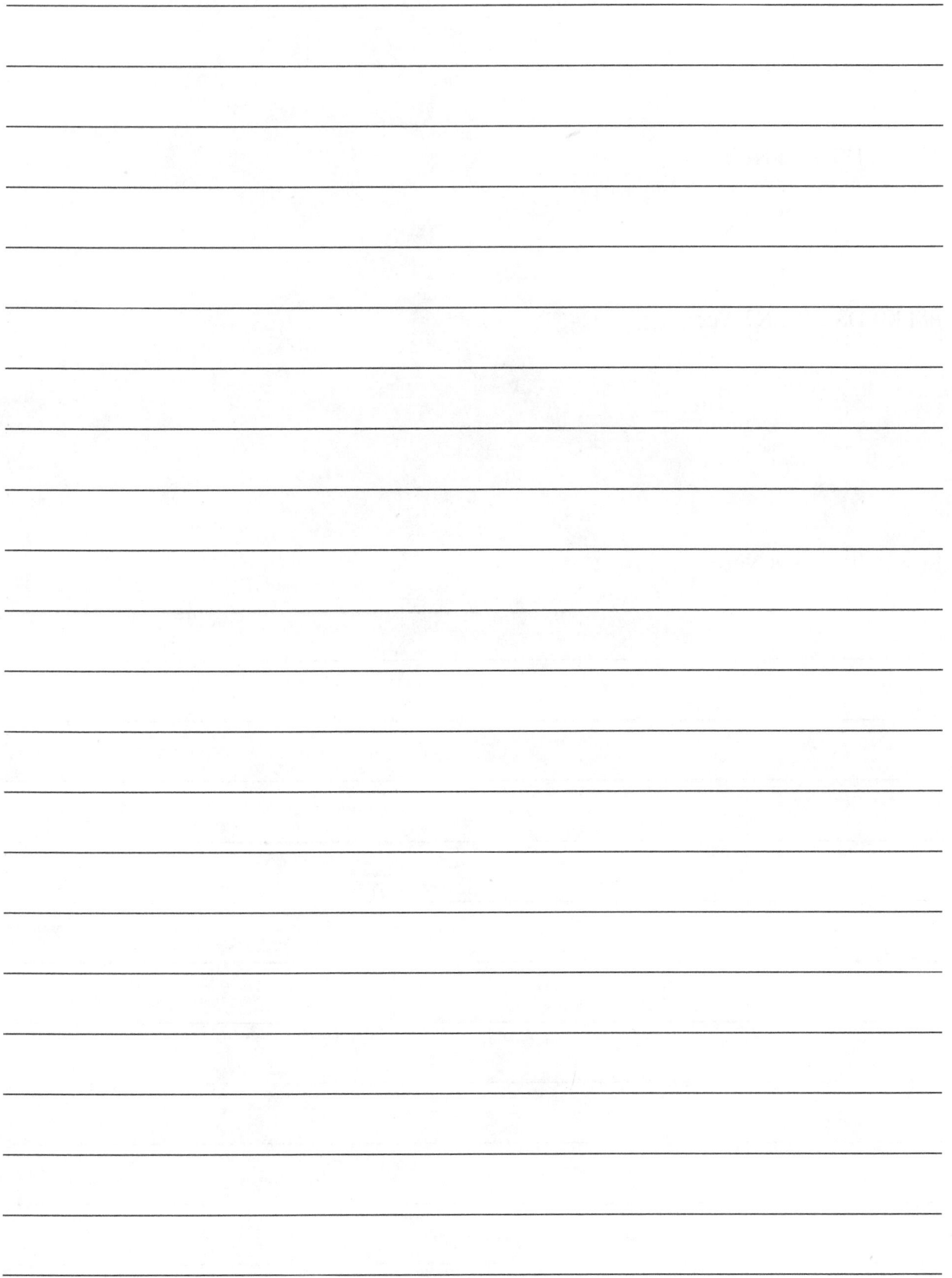

Date_____   Patient ID_____   Room Number_____

Medications   Administering   Mathematical

Instructions   Computations

EST	Military	Notes	EST	Military	Notes	EST	Military	Notes	EST	Military	Notes
8:00 AM	08:00		3:15PM	15:15		10:15PM	22:15		5:15AM	05:15	
8:15 AM	08:15		3:30PM	15:30		10:30PM	22:30		5:30AM	05:30	
8:30AM	08:30		3:45PM	15:45		10:45PM	22:45		5:45AM	05:45	
8:45AM	08:45		4:00PM	16:00		11:00PM	23:00		6:00AM	06:00	
9:00AM	09:00		4:15PM	16:15		11:15PM	23:15		6:15AM	06:15	
9:15AM	09:15		4:30PM	16:30		11:30PM	23:30		6:30AM	06:30	
9:30AM	09:30		4:45PM	16:45		11:45PM	23:45		6:45AM	06:45	
9:45AM	09:45		5:00PM	17:00		12:00AM	24:00		7:00AM	07:00	
10:00AM	10:00		5:15PM	17:15		12:15AM	24:15		7:15AM	07:15	
10:15AM	10:15		5:30PM	17:30		12:30AM	24:30		730AM	07:30	
10:30AM	10:30		5:45PM	17:45		12:45AM	24:45		7:45AM	07:45	
10:45AM	10:45		6:00PM	18:00		1:00AM	01:00				
11:00AM	11:00		6:15PM	18:15		1:15AM	01:15				
11:15AM	11:15		6:30PM	18:30		1:30AM	01:30				
11:30AM	11:30		6:45PM	18:45		1:45AM	01:45				
11:45AM	11:45		7:00PM	19:00		2:00AM	02:00				
12:00PM	12:00		7:15PM	19:15		2:15AM	02:15				
12:15PM	12:15		7:30PM	19:30		2:45AM	02:45				
12:30PM	12:30		7:45PM	19:45		3:00AM	03:00				
12:45PM	12:45		8:00PM	20:00		3:15AM	03:15				
1:00PM	13:00		8:15PM	20:15		3:30AM	03:30				
1:15PM	13:15		8:30PM	20:30		3:45AM	03:45				
1:30PM	13:30		8:45PM	20:45		4:00AM	04:00				
1:45PM	13:45		9:00PM	21:00		4:15AM	04:15				
2:00PM	14:00		9:15PM	21:15		4:30AM	04:30				
2:15PM	14:15		9:30PM	21:30		4:45AM	04:45				
2:30PM	14:30		9:45PM	21:45		5:00AM	05:00				
2:45PM	14:45		10:00PM	22:00							
3:00PM	15:00										

Date_____ Patient ID_____ Room Number_____

AM MEDS GIVEN? Yes_____

No_____

PM MEDS GIVEN? Yes_____

No_____

Results/Progress Notes:

_____

_____

_____

_____

_____

_____

_____

_____

_____

_____

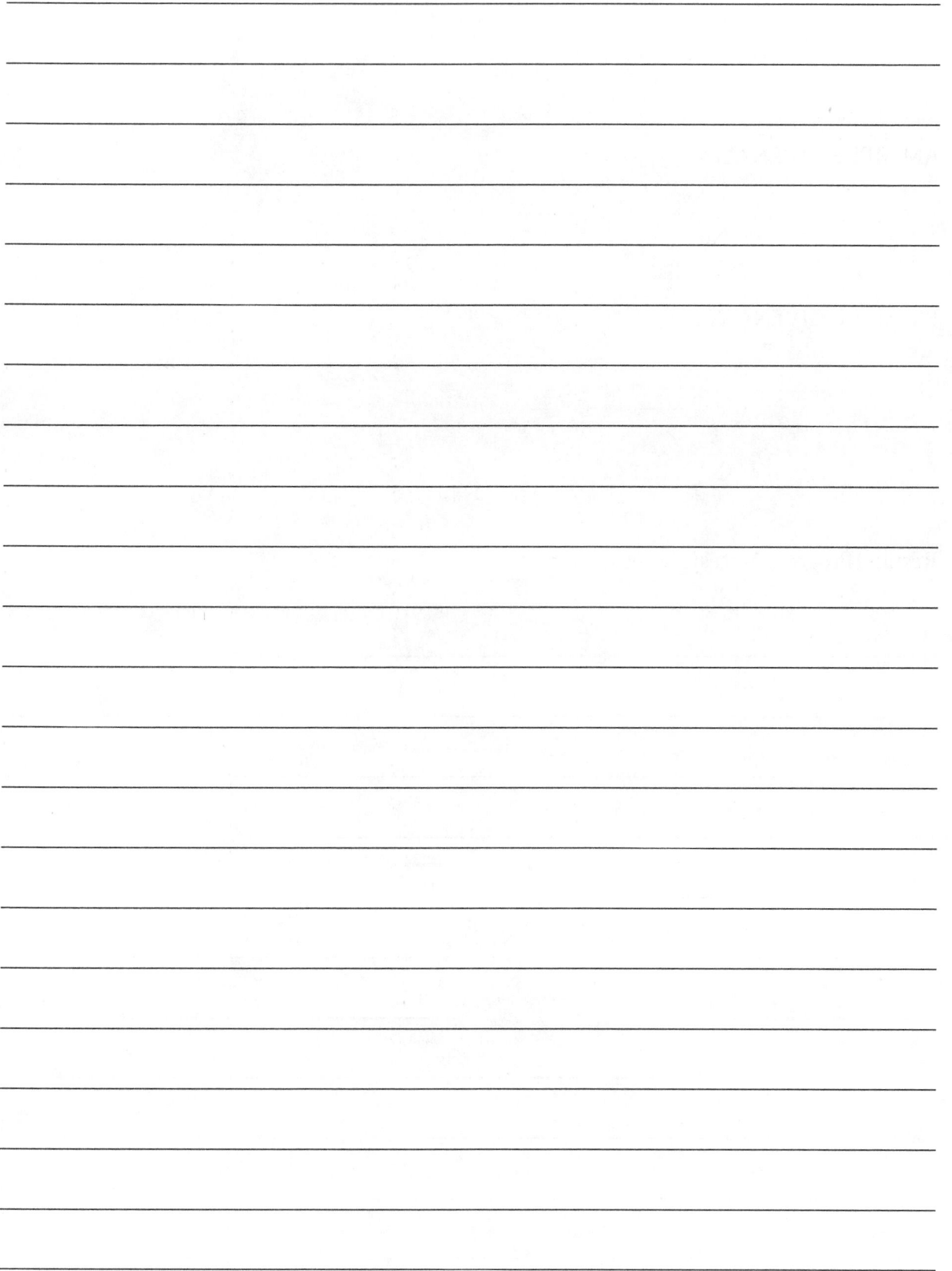

Date_____ Patient ID_____ Room Number_____

Medications	Administering Instructions

Mathematical Computations

EST	Military	Notes	EST	Military	Notes	EST	Military	Notes	EST	Military	Notes
8:00 AM	08:00		3:15PM	15:15		10:15PM	22:15		5:15AM	05:15	
8:15 AM	08:15		3:30PM	15:30		10:30PM	22:30		5:30AM	05:30	
8:30AM	08:30		3:45PM	15:45		10:45PM	22:45		5:45AM	05:45	
8:45AM	08:45		4:00PM	16:00		11:00PM	23:00		6:00AM	06:00	
9:00AM	09:00		4:15PM	16:15		11:15PM	23:15		6:15AM	06:15	
9:15AM	09:15		4:30PM	16:30		11:30PM	23:30		6:30AM	06:30	
9:30AM	09:30		4:45PM	16:45		11:45PM	23:45		6:45AM	06:45	
9:45AM	09:45		5:00PM	17:00		12:00AM	24:00		7:00AM	07:00	
10:00AM	10:00		5:15PM	17:15		12:15AM	24:15		7:15AM	07:15	
10:15AM	10:15		5:30PM	17:30		12:30AM	24:30		730AM	07:30	
10:30AM	10:30		5:45PM	17:45		12:45AM	24:45		7:45AM	07:45	
10:45AM	10:45		6:00PM	18:00		1:00AM	01:00				
11:00AM	11:00		6:15PM	18:15		1:15AM	01:15				
11:15AM	11:15		6:30PM	18:30		1:30AM	01:30				
11:30AM	11:30		6:45PM	18:45		1:45AM	01:45				
11:45AM	11:45		7:00PM	19:00		2:00AM	02:00				
12:00PM	12:00		7:15PM	19:15		2:15AM	02:15				
12:15PM	12:15		7:30PM	19:30		2:45AM	02:45				
12:30PM	12:30		7:45PM	19:45		3:00AM	03:00				
12:45PM	12:45		8:00PM	20:00		3:15AM	03:15				
1:00PM	13:00		8:15PM	20:15		3:30AM	03:30				
1:15PM	13:15		8:30PM	20:30		3:45AM	03:45				
1:30PM	13:30		8:45PM	20:45		4:00AM	04:00				
1:45PM	13:45		9:00PM	21:00		4:15AM	04:15				
2:00PM	14:00		9:15PM	21:15		4:30AM	04:30				
2:15PM	14:15		9:30PM	21:30		4:45AM	04:45				
2:30PM	14:30		9:45PM	21:45		5:00AM	05:00				
2:45PM	14:45		10:00PM	22:00							
3:00PM	15:00										

Date_____   Patient ID_____   Room Number_____

AM MEDS GIVEN? Yes_____

No_____

PM MEDS GIVEN? Yes_____

No_____

Results/Progress Notes:

_____

_____

_____

_____

_____

_____

_____

_____

_____

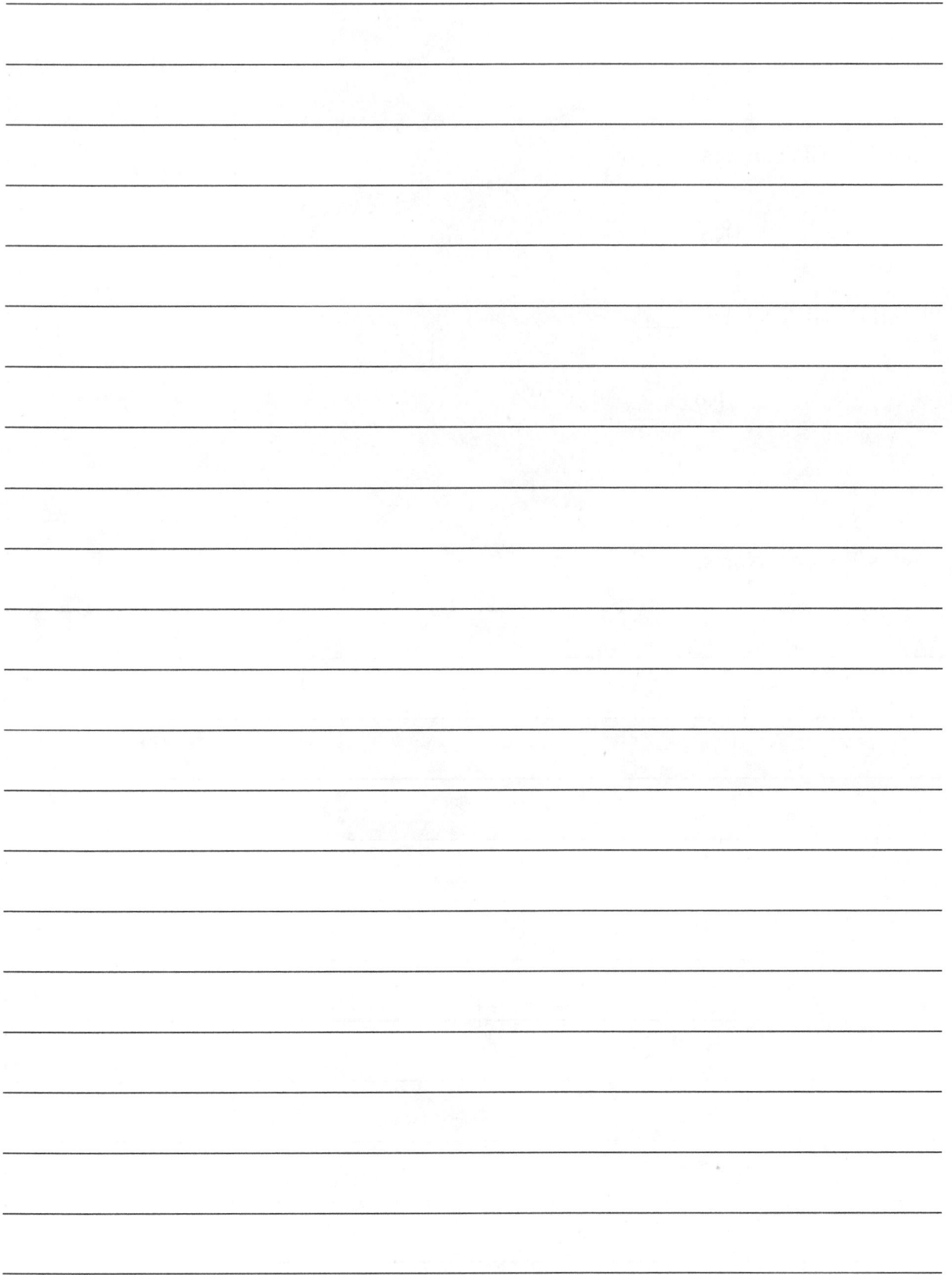

Date_____ Patient ID_____ Room Number_____

Medications

Administering

Instructions

Mathematical

Computations

EST	Military	Notes	EST	Military	Notes	EST	Military	Notes	EST	Military	Notes
8:00 AM	08:00		3:15PM	15:15		10:15PM	22:15		5:15AM	05:15	
8:15 AM	08:15		3:30PM	15:30		10:30PM	22:30		5:30AM	05:30	
8:30AM	08:30		3:45PM	15:45		10:45PM	22:45		5:45AM	05:45	
8:45AM	08:45		4:00PM	16:00		11:00PM	23:00		6:00AM	06:00	
9:00AM	09:00		4:15PM	16:15		11:15PM	23:15		6:15AM	06:15	
9:15AM	09:15		4:30PM	16:30		11:30PM	23:30		6:30AM	06:30	
9:30AM	09:30		4:45PM	16:45		11:45PM	23:45		6:45AM	06:45	
9:45AM	09:45		5:00PM	17:00		12:00AM	24:00		7:00AM	07:00	
10:00AM	10:00		5:15PM	17:15		12:15AM	24:15		7:15AM	07:15	
10:15AM	10:15		5:30PM	17:30		12:30AM	24:30		730AM	07:30	
10:30AM	10:30		5:45PM	17:45		12:45AM	24:45		7:45AM	07:45	
10:45AM	10:45		6:00PM	18:00		1:00AM	01:00				
11:00AM	11:00		6:15PM	18:15		1:15AM	01:15				
11:15AM	11:15		6:30PM	18:30		1:30AM	01:30				
11:30AM	11:30		6:45PM	18:45		1:45AM	01:45				
11:45AM	11:45		7:00PM	19:00		2:00AM	02:00				
12:00PM	12:00		7:15PM	19:15		2:15AM	02:15				
12:15PM	12:15		7:30PM	19:30		2:45AM	02:45				
12:30PM	12:30		7:45PM	19:45		3:00AM	03:00				
12:45PM	12:45		8:00PM	20:00		3:15AM	03:15				
1:00PM	13:00		8:15PM	20:15		3:30AM	03:30				
1:15PM	13:15		8:30PM	20:30		3:45AM	03:45				
1:30PM	13:30		8:45PM	20:45		4:00AM	04:00				
1:45PM	13:45		9:00PM	21:00		4:15AM	04:15				
2:00PM	14:00		9:15PM	21:15		4:30AM	04:30				
2:15PM	14:15		9:30PM	21:30		4:45AM	04:45				
2:30PM	14:30		9:45PM	21:45		5:00AM	05:00				
2:45PM	14:45		10:00PM	22:00							
3:00PM	15:00										

Date_____   Patient ID_____   Room Number_____

AM MEDS GIVEN? Yes_____

                  No_____

PM MEDS GIVEN? Yes_____

                  No_____

Results/Progress Notes:

_____

_____

_____

_____

_____

_____

_____

_____

_____

_____

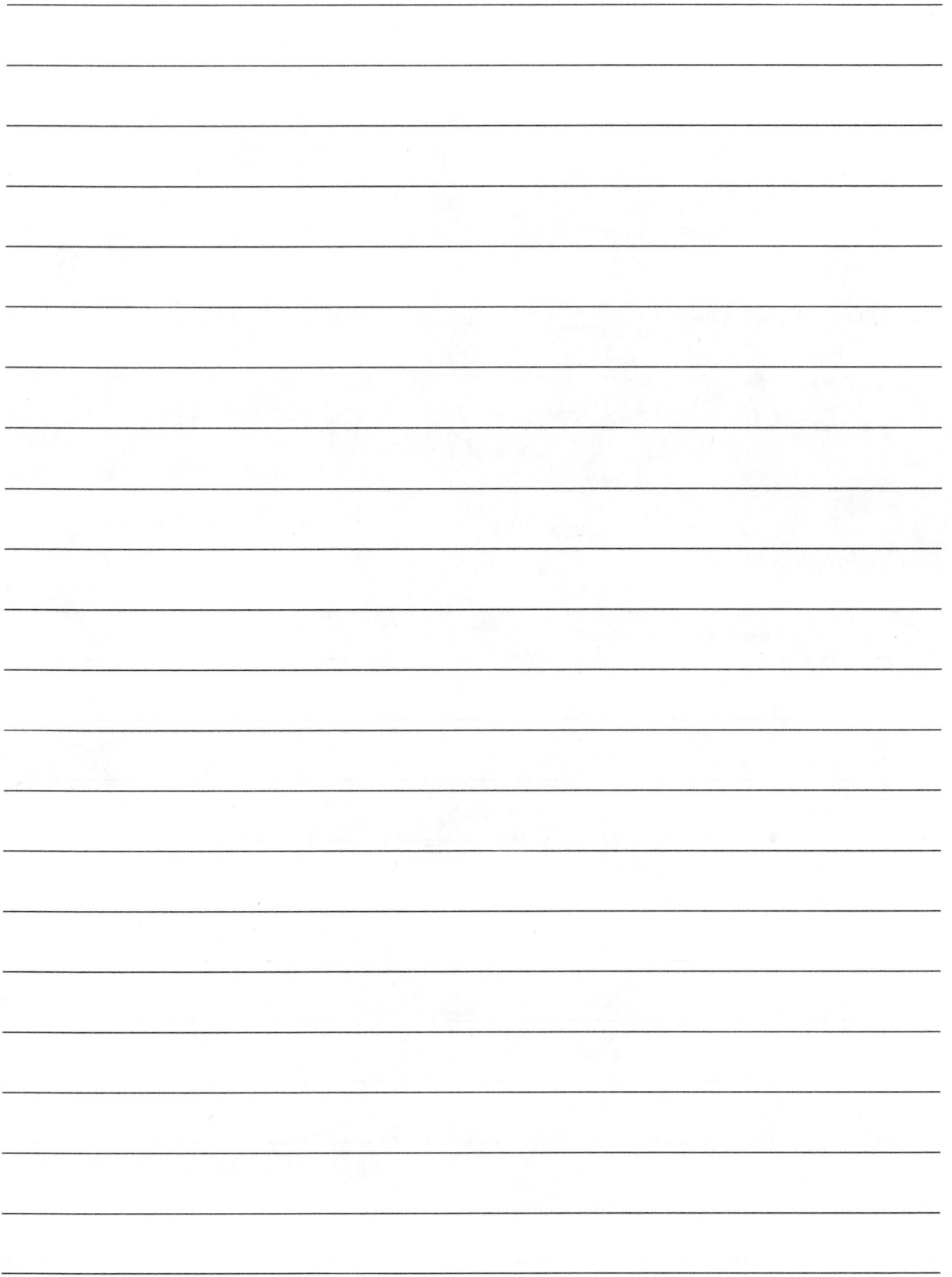

Date_____   Patient ID_____   Room Number_____

Medications   Administering   Mathematical

Instructions   Computations

EST	Military	Notes	EST	Military	Notes	EST	Military	Notes	EST	Military	Notes
8:00 AM	08:00		3:15PM	15:15		10:15PM	22:15		5:15AM	05:15	
8:15 AM	08:15		3:30PM	15:30		10:30PM	22:30		5:30AM	05:30	
8:30AM	08:30		3:45PM	15:45		10:45PM	22:45		5:45AM	05:45	
8:45AM	08:45		4:00PM	16:00		11:00PM	23:00		6:00AM	06:00	
9:00AM	09:00		4:15PM	16:15		11:15PM	23:15		6:15AM	06:15	
9:15AM	09:15		4:30PM	16:30		11:30PM	23:30		6:30AM	06:30	
9:30AM	09:30		4:45PM	16:45		11:45PM	23:45		6:45AM	06:45	
9:45AM	09:45		5:00PM	17:00		12:00AM	24:00		7:00AM	07:00	
10:00AM	10:00		5:15PM	17:15		12:15AM	24:15		7:15AM	07:15	
10:15AM	10:15		5:30PM	17:30		12:30AM	24:30		730AM	07:30	
10:30AM	10:30		5:45PM	17:45		12:45AM	24:45		7:45AM	07:45	
10:45AM	10:45		6:00PM	18:00		1:00AM	01:00				
11:00AM	11:00		6:15PM	18:15		1:15AM	01:15				
11:15AM	11:15		6:30PM	18:30		1:30AM	01:30				
11:30AM	11:30		6:45PM	18:45		1:45AM	01:45				
11:45AM	11:45		7:00PM	19:00		2:00AM	02:00				
12:00PM	12:00		7:15PM	19:15		2:15AM	02:15				
12:15PM	12:15		7:30PM	19:30		2:45AM	02:45				
12:30PM	12:30		7:45PM	19:45		3:00AM	03:00				
12:45PM	12:45		8:00PM	20:00		3:15AM	03:15				
1:00PM	13:00		8:15PM	20:15		3:30AM	03:30				
1:15PM	13:15		8:30PM	20:30		3:45AM	03:45				
1:30PM	13:30		8:45PM	20:45		4:00AM	04:00				
1:45PM	13:45		9:00PM	21:00		4:15AM	04:15				
2:00PM	14:00		9:15PM	21:15		4:30AM	04:30				
2:15PM	14:15		9:30PM	21:30		4:45AM	04:45				
2:30PM	14:30		9:45PM	21:45		5:00AM	05:00				
2:45PM	14:45		10:00PM	22:00							
3:00PM	15:00										

Date_____ Patient ID_____ Room Number_____

AM MEDS GIVEN? Yes_____

      No_____

PM MEDS GIVEN? Yes_____

      No_____

Results/Progress Notes:

_____

_____

_____

_____

_____

_____

_____

_____

_____

_____

Date_____ Patient ID_____ Room Number_____

Medications   Administering   Mathematical

                     Instructions   Computations

Medications	Administering Instructions	Mathematical Computations

EST	Military	Notes	EST	Military	Notes	EST	Military	Notes	EST	Military	Notes
8:00 AM	08:00		3:15PM	15:15		10:15PM	22:15		5:15AM	05:15	
8:15 AM	08:15		3:30PM	15:30		10:30PM	22:30		5:30AM	05:30	
8:30AM	08:30		3:45PM	15:45		10:45PM	22:45		5:45AM	05:45	
8:45AM	08:45		4:00PM	16:00		11:00PM	23:00		6:00AM	06:00	
9:00AM	09:00		4:15PM	16:15		11:15PM	23:15		6:15AM	06:15	
9:15AM	09:15		4:30PM	16:30		11:30PM	23:30		6:30AM	06:30	
9:30AM	09:30		4:45PM	16:45		11:45PM	23:45		6:45AM	06:45	
9:45AM	09:45		5:00PM	17:00		12:00AM	24:00		7:00AM	07:00	
10:00AM	10:00		5:15PM	17:15		12:15AM	24:15		7:15AM	07:15	
10:15AM	10:15		5:30PM	17:30		12:30AM	24:30		730AM	07:30	
10:30AM	10:30		5:45PM	17:45		12:45AM	24:45		7:45AM	07:45	
10:45AM	10:45		6:00PM	18:00		1:00AM	01:00				
11:00AM	11:00		6:15PM	18:15		1:15AM	01:15				
11:15AM	11:15		6:30PM	18:30		1:30AM	01:30				
11:30AM	11:30		6:45PM	18:45		1:45AM	01:45				
11:45AM	11:45		7:00PM	19:00		2:00AM	02:00				
12:00PM	12:00		7:15PM	19:15		2:15AM	02:15				
12:15PM	12:15		7:30PM	19:30		2:45AM	02:45				
12:30PM	12:30		7:45PM	19:45		3:00AM	03:00				
12:45PM	12:45		8:00PM	20:00		3:15AM	03:15				
1:00PM	13:00		8:15PM	20:15		3:30AM	03:30				
1:15PM	13:15		8:30PM	20:30		3:45AM	03:45				
1:30PM	13:30		8:45PM	20:45		4:00AM	04:00				
1:45PM	13:45		9:00PM	21:00		4:15AM	04:15				
2:00PM	14:00		9:15PM	21:15		4:30AM	04:30				
2:15PM	14:15		9:30PM	21:30		4:45AM	04:45				
2:30PM	14:30		9:45PM	21:45		5:00AM	05:00				
2:45PM	14:45		10:00PM	22:00							
3:00PM	15:00										

Date_____   Patient ID_____   Room Number_____

AM MEDS GIVEN? Yes_____

No_____

PM MEDS GIVEN? Yes_____

No_____

Results/Progress Notes:

_____

_____

_____

_____

_____

_____

_____

_____

_____

_____

_____

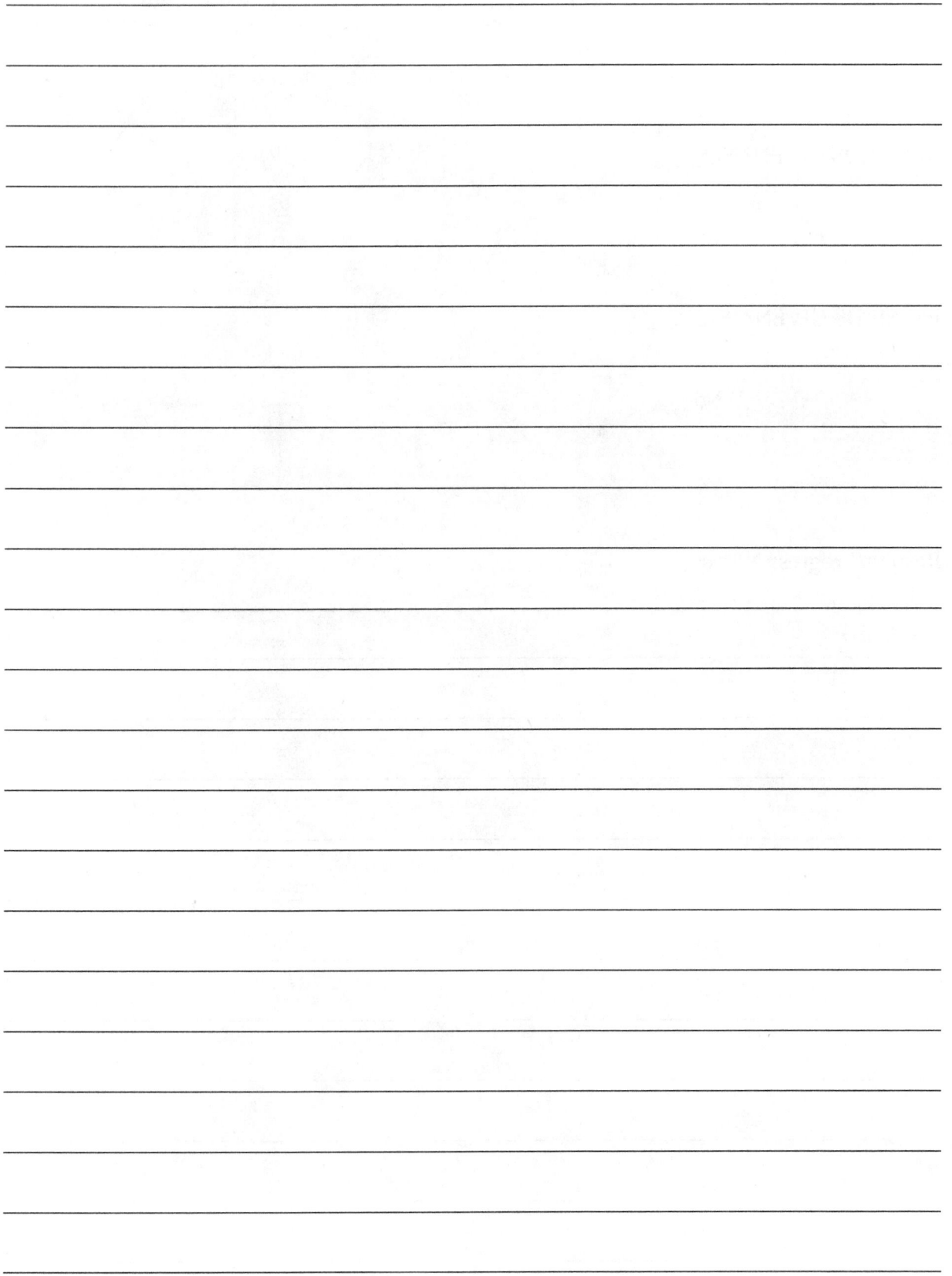

Date_____ Patient ID_____ Room Number_____

Medications	Administering Instructions	Mathematical Computations

EST	Military	Notes	EST	Military	Notes	EST	Military	Notes	EST	Military	Notes
8:00 AM	08:00		3:15PM	15:15		10:15PM	22:15		5:15AM	05:15	
8:15 AM	08:15		3:30PM	15:30		10:30PM	22:30		5:30AM	05:30	
8:30AM	08:30		3:45PM	15:45		10:45PM	22:45		5:45AM	05:45	
8:45AM	08:45		4:00PM	16:00		11:00PM	23:00		6:00AM	06:00	
9:00AM	09:00		4:15PM	16:15		11:15PM	23:15		6:15AM	06:15	
9:15AM	09:15		4:30PM	16:30		11:30PM	23:30		6:30AM	06:30	
9:30AM	09:30		4:45PM	16:45		11:45PM	23:45		6:45AM	06:45	
9:45AM	09:45		5:00PM	17:00		12:00AM	24:00		7:00AM	07:00	
10:00AM	10:00		5:15PM	17:15		12:15AM	24:15		7:15AM	07:15	
10:15AM	10:15		5:30PM	17:30		12:30AM	24:30		730AM	07:30	
10:30AM	10:30		5:45PM	17:45		12:45AM	24:45		7:45AM	07:45	
10:45AM	10:45		6:00PM	18:00		1:00AM	01:00				
11:00AM	11:00		6:15PM	18:15		1:15AM	01:15				
11:15AM	11:15		6:30PM	18:30		1:30AM	01:30				
11:30AM	11:30		6:45PM	18:45		1:45AM	01:45				
11:45AM	11:45		7:00PM	19:00		2:00AM	02:00				
12:00PM	12:00		7:15PM	19:15		2:15AM	02:15				
12:15PM	12:15		7:30PM	19:30		2:45AM	02:45				
12:30PM	12:30		7:45PM	19:45		3:00AM	03:00				
12:45PM	12:45		8:00PM	20:00		3:15AM	03:15				
1:00PM	13:00		8:15PM	20:15		3:30AM	03:30				
1:15PM	13:15		8:30PM	20:30		3:45AM	03:45				
1:30PM	13:30		8:45PM	20:45		4:00AM	04:00				
1:45PM	13:45		9:00PM	21:00		4:15AM	04:15				
2:00PM	14:00		9:15PM	21:15		4:30AM	04:30				
2:15PM	14:15		9:30PM	21:30		4:45AM	04:45				
2:30PM	14:30		9:45PM	21:45		5:00AM	05:00				
2:45PM	14:45		10:00PM	22:00							
3:00PM	15:00										

Date_____   Patient ID_____   Room Number_____

AM MEDS GIVEN? Yes_____

            No_____

PM MEDS GIVEN? Yes_____

            No_____

Results/Progress Notes:

_____

_____

_____

_____

_____

_____

_____

_____

_____

_____

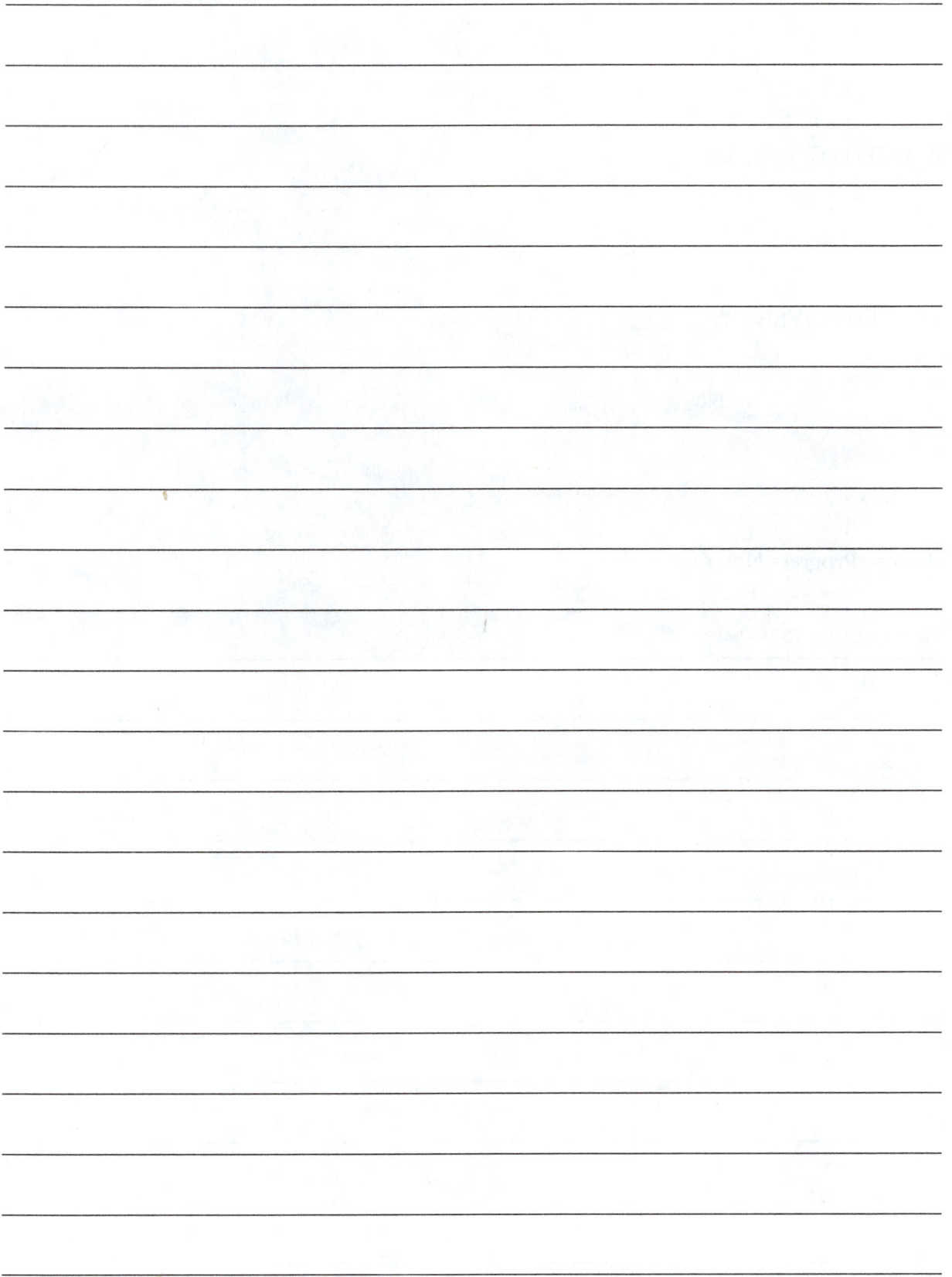

Date_____ Patient ID_____ Room Number_____

Medications   Administering   Mathematical

                     Instructions   Computations

EST	Military	Notes	EST	Military	Notes	EST	Military	Notes	EST	Military	Notes
8:00 AM	08:00		3:15PM	15:15		10:15PM	22:15		5:15AM	05:15	
8:15 AM	08:15		3:30PM	15:30		10:30PM	22:30		5:30AM	05:30	
8:30AM	08:30		3:45PM	15:45		10:45PM	22:45		5:45AM	05:45	
8:45AM	08:45		4:00PM	16:00		11:00PM	23:00		6:00AM	06:00	
9:00AM	09:00		4:15PM	16:15		11:15PM	23:15		6:15AM	06:15	
9:15AM	09:15		4:30PM	16:30		11:30PM	23:30		6:30AM	06:30	
9:30AM	09:30		4:45PM	16:45		11:45PM	23:45		6:45AM	06:45	
9:45AM	09:45		5:00PM	17:00		12:00AM	24:00		7:00AM	07:00	
10:00AM	10:00		5:15PM	17:15		12:15AM	24:15		7:15AM	07:15	
10:15AM	10:15		5:30PM	17:30		12:30AM	24:30		730AM	07:30	
10:30AM	10:30		5:45PM	17:45		12:45AM	24:45		7:45AM	07:45	
10:45AM	10:45		6:00PM	18:00		1:00AM	01:00				
11:00AM	11:00		6:15PM	18:15		1:15AM	01:15				
11:15AM	11:15		6:30PM	18:30		1:30AM	01:30				
11:30AM	11:30		6:45PM	18:45		1:45AM	01:45				
11:45AM	11:45		7:00PM	19:00		2:00AM	02:00				
12:00PM	12:00		7:15PM	19:15		2:15AM	02:15				
12:15PM	12:15		7:30PM	19:30		2:45AM	02:45				
12:30PM	12:30		7:45PM	19:45		3:00AM	03:00				
12:45PM	12:45		8:00PM	20:00		3:15AM	03:15				
1:00PM	13:00		8:15PM	20:15		3:30AM	03:30				
1:15PM	13:15		8:30PM	20:30		3:45AM	03:45				
1:30PM	13:30		8:45PM	20:45		4:00AM	04:00				
1:45PM	13:45		9:00PM	21:00		4:15AM	04:15				
2:00PM	14:00		9:15PM	21:15		4:30AM	04:30				
2:15PM	14:15		9:30PM	21:30		4:45AM	04:45				
2:30PM	14:30		9:45PM	21:45		5:00AM	05:00				
2:45PM	14:45		10:00PM	22:00							
3:00PM	15:00										

Date_____   Patient ID_____   Room Number_____

AM MEDS GIVEN? Yes_____

                       No_____

PM MEDS GIVEN? Yes_____

                       No_____

Results/Progress Notes:

_____

_____

_____

_____

_____

_____

_____

_____

_____

_____

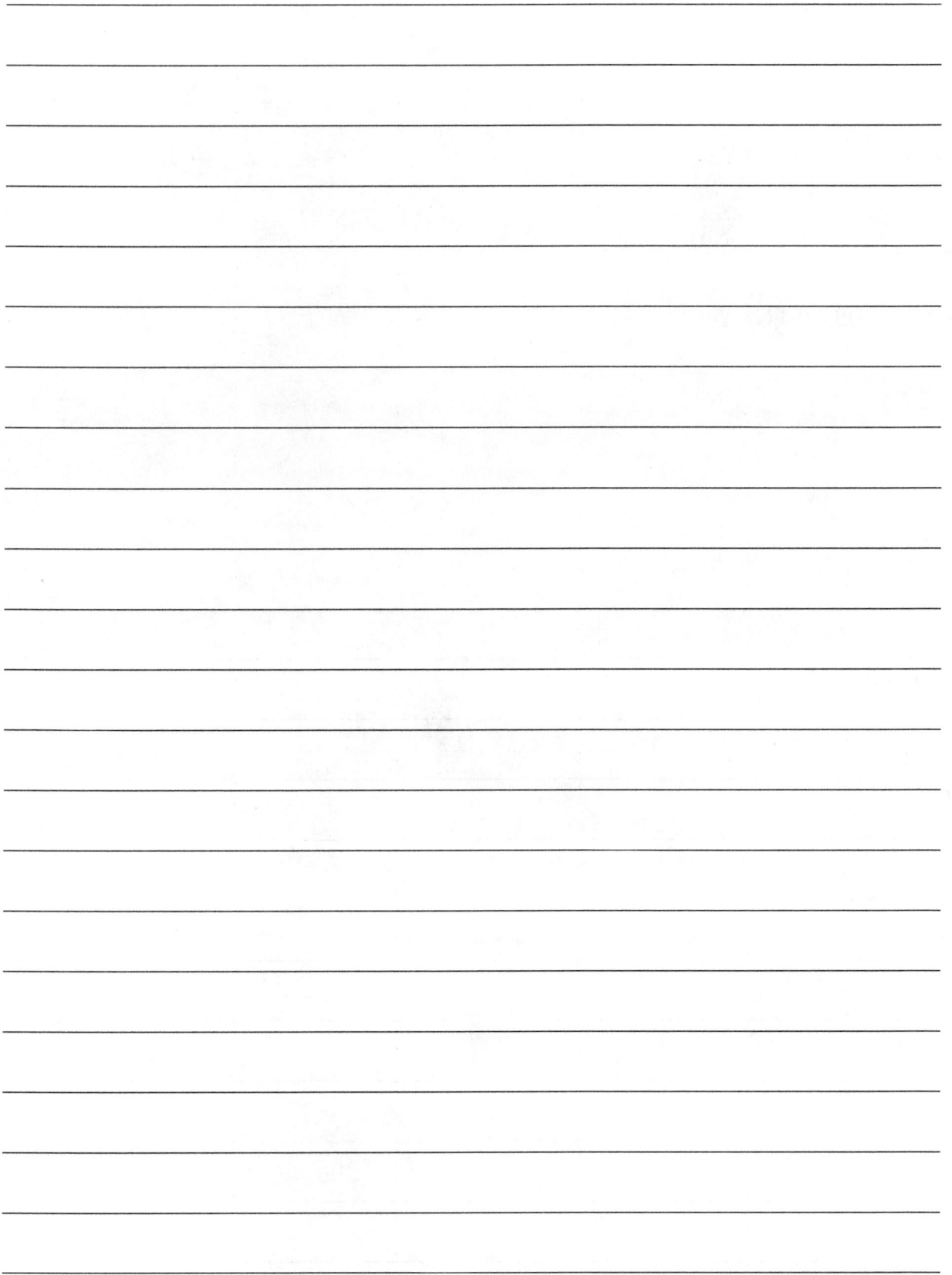

Date_____ Patient ID_____ Room Number_____

Medications	Administering Instructions	Mathematical Computations

EST	Military	Notes	EST	Military	Notes	EST	Military	Notes	EST	Military	Notes
8:00 AM	08:00		3:15PM	15:15		10:15PM	22:15		5:15AM	05:15	
8:15 AM	08:15		3:30PM	15:30		10:30PM	22:30		5:30AM	05:30	
8:30AM	08:30		3:45PM	15:45		10:45PM	22:45		5:45AM	05:45	
8:45AM	08:45		4:00PM	16:00		11:00PM	23:00		6:00AM	06:00	
9:00AM	09:00		4:15PM	16:15		11:15PM	23:15		6:15AM	06:15	
9:15AM	09:15		4:30PM	16:30		11:30PM	23:30		6:30AM	06:30	
9:30AM	09:30		4:45PM	16:45		11:45PM	23:45		6:45AM	06:45	
9:45AM	09:45		5:00PM	17:00		12:00AM	24:00		7:00AM	07:00	
10:00AM	10:00		5:15PM	17:15		12:15AM	24:15		7:15AM	07:15	
10:15AM	10:15		5:30PM	17:30		12:30AM	24:30		730AM	07:30	
10:30AM	10:30		5:45PM	17:45		12:45AM	24:45		7:45AM	07:45	
10:45AM	10:45		6:00PM	18:00		1:00AM	01:00				
11:00AM	11:00		6:15PM	18:15		1:15AM	01:15				
11:15AM	11:15		6:30PM	18:30		1:30AM	01:30				
11:30AM	11:30		6:45PM	18:45		1:45AM	01:45				
11:45AM	11:45		7:00PM	19:00		2:00AM	02:00				
12:00PM	12:00		7:15PM	19:15		2:15AM	02:15				
12:15PM	12:15		7:30PM	19:30		2:45AM	02:45				
12:30PM	12:30		7:45PM	19:45		3:00AM	03:00				
12:45PM	12:45		8:00PM	20:00		3:15AM	03:15				
1:00PM	13:00		8:15PM	20:15		3:30AM	03:30				
1:15PM	13:15		8:30PM	20:30		3:45AM	03:45				
1:30PM	13:30		8:45PM	20:45		4:00AM	04:00				
1:45PM	13:45		9:00PM	21:00		4:15AM	04:15				
2:00PM	14:00		9:15PM	21:15		4:30AM	04:30				
2:15PM	14:15		9:30PM	21:30		4:45AM	04:45				
2:30PM	14:30		9:45PM	21:45		5:00AM	05:00				
2:45PM	14:45		10:00PM	22:00							
3:00PM	15:00										

Date_____ Patient ID_____ Room Number_____

AM MEDS GIVEN? Yes_____

No_____

PM MEDS GIVEN? Yes_____

No_____

Results/Progress Notes:

_____

_____

_____

_____

_____

_____

_____

_____

_____

_____

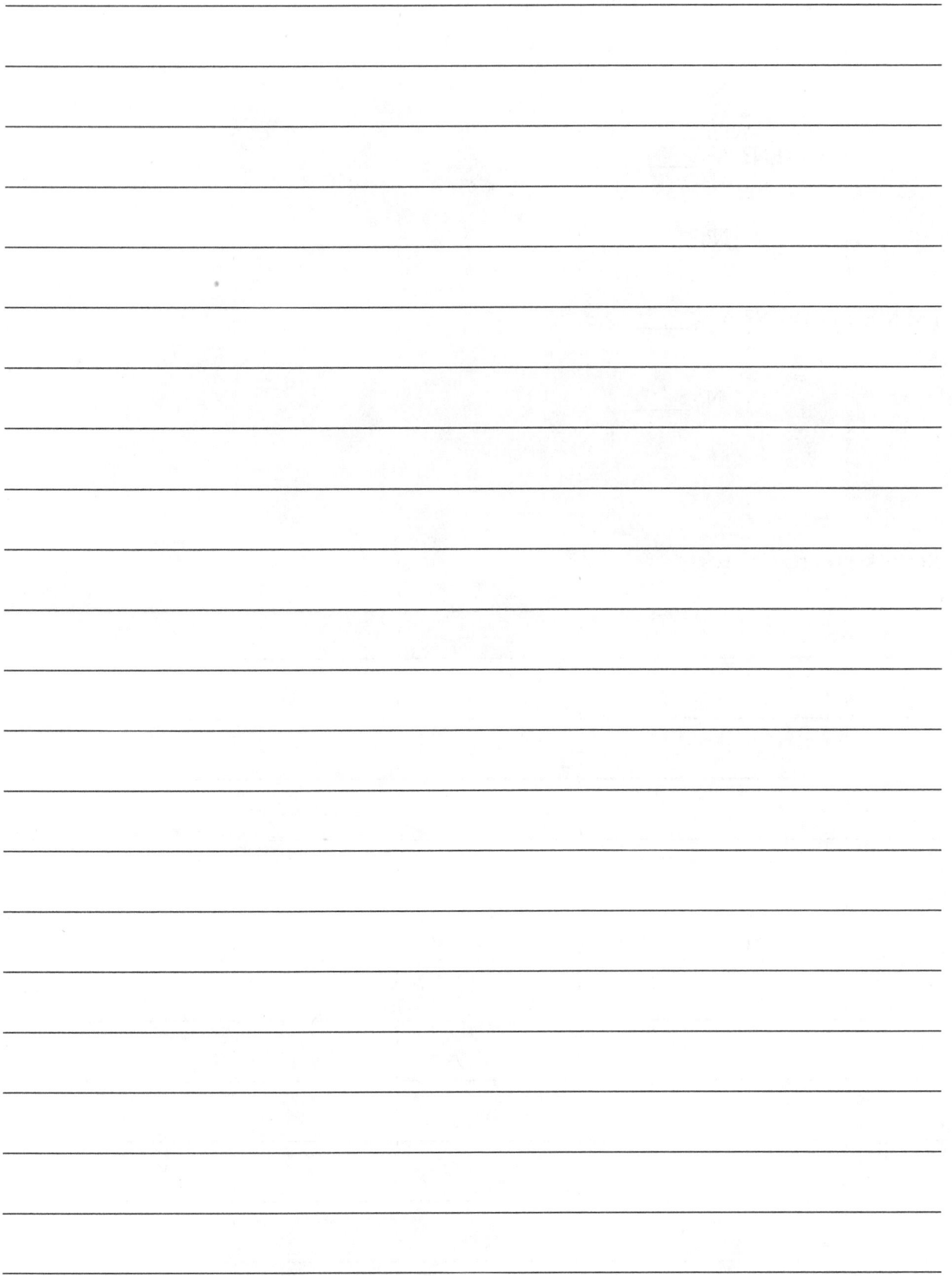

Date_____ Patient ID_____ Room Number_____

Medications	Administering Instructions	Mathematical Computations

EST	Military	Notes	EST	Military	Notes	EST	Military	Notes	EST	Military	Notes
8:00 AM	08:00		3:15PM	15:15		10:15PM	22:15		5:15AM	05:15	
8:15 AM	08:15		3:30PM	15:30		10:30PM	22:30		5:30AM	05:30	
8:30AM	08:30		3:45PM	15:45		10:45PM	22:45		5:45AM	05:45	
8:45AM	08:45		4:00PM	16:00		11:00PM	23:00		6:00AM	06:00	
9:00AM	09:00		4:15PM	16:15		11:15PM	23:15		6:15AM	06:15	
9:15AM	09:15		4:30PM	16:30		11:30PM	23:30		6:30AM	06:30	
9:30AM	09:30		4:45PM	16:45		11:45PM	23:45		6:45AM	06:45	
9:45AM	09:45		5:00PM	17:00		12:00AM	24:00		7:00AM	07:00	
10:00AM	10:00		5:15PM	17:15		12:15AM	24:15		7:15AM	07:15	
10:15AM	10:15		5:30PM	17:30		12:30AM	24:30		730AM	07:30	
10:30AM	10:30		5:45PM	17:45		12:45AM	24:45		7:45AM	07:45	
10:45AM	10:45		6:00PM	18:00		1:00AM	01:00				
11:00AM	11:00		6:15PM	18:15		1:15AM	01:15				
11:15AM	11:15		6:30PM	18:30		1:30AM	01:30				
11:30AM	11:30		6:45PM	18:45		1:45AM	01:45				
11:45AM	11:45		7:00PM	19:00		2:00AM	02:00				
12:00PM	12:00		7:15PM	19:15		2:15AM	02:15				
12:15PM	12:15		7:30PM	19:30		2:45AM	02:45				
12:30PM	12:30		7:45PM	19:45		3:00AM	03:00				
12:45PM	12:45		8:00PM	20:00		3:15AM	03:15				
1:00PM	13:00		8:15PM	20:15		3:30AM	03:30				
1:15PM	13:15		8:30PM	20:30		3:45AM	03:45				
1:30PM	13:30		8:45PM	20:45		4:00AM	04:00				
1:45PM	13:45		9:00PM	21:00		4:15AM	04:15				
2:00PM	14:00		9:15PM	21:15		4:30AM	04:30				
2:15PM	14:15		9:30PM	21:30		4:45AM	04:45				
2:30PM	14:30		9:45PM	21:45		5:00AM	05:00				
2:45PM	14:45		10:00PM	22:00							
3:00PM	15:00										

Date_____   Patient ID_____   Room Number_____

AM MEDS GIVEN? Yes_____

No_____

PM MEDS GIVEN? Yes_____

No_____

Results/Progress Notes:

_____

_____

_____

_____

_____

_____

_____

_____

_____

_____

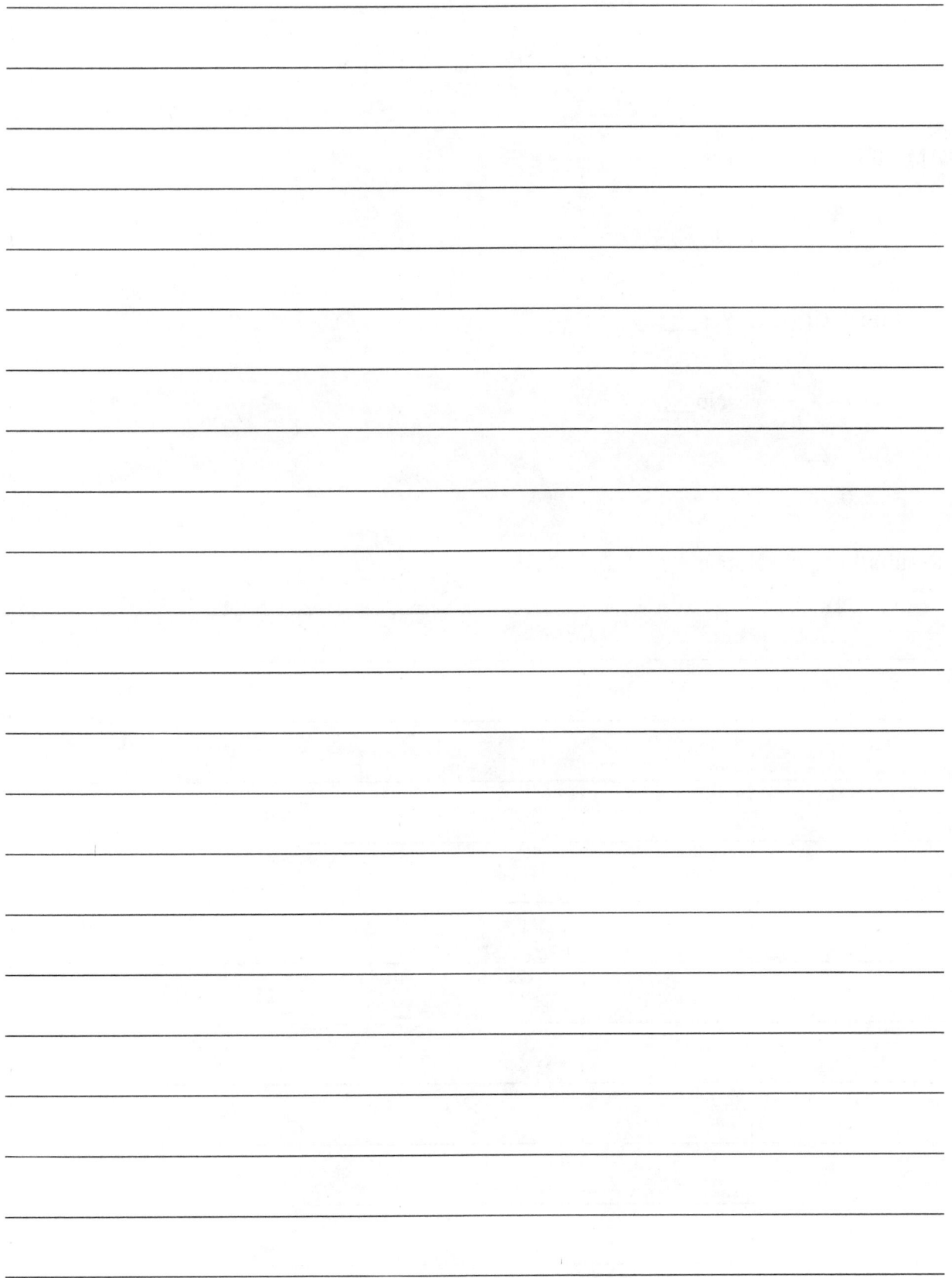

Date_____ Patient ID_____ Room Number_____

Medications	Administering Instructions

Mathematical Computations

EST	Military	Notes	EST	Military	Notes	EST	Military	Notes	EST	Military	Notes
8:00 AM	08:00		3:15PM	15:15		10:15PM	22:15		5:15AM	05:15	
8:15 AM	08:15		3:30PM	15:30		10:30PM	22:30		5:30AM	05:30	
8:30AM	08:30		3:45PM	15:45		10:45PM	22:45		5:45AM	05:45	
8:45AM	08:45		4:00PM	16:00		11:00PM	23:00		6:00AM	06:00	
9:00AM	09:00		4:15PM	16:15		11:15PM	23:15		6:15AM	06:15	
9:15AM	09:15		4:30PM	16:30		11:30PM	23:30		6:30AM	06:30	
9:30AM	09:30		4:45PM	16:45		11:45PM	23:45		6:45AM	06:45	
9:45AM	09:45		5:00PM	17:00		12:00AM	24:00		7:00AM	07:00	
10:00AM	10:00		5:15PM	17:15		12:15AM	24:15		7:15AM	07:15	
10:15AM	10:15		5:30PM	17:30		12:30AM	24:30		730AM	07:30	
10:30AM	10:30		5:45PM	17:45		12:45AM	24:45		7:45AM	07:45	
10:45AM	10:45		6:00PM	18:00		1:00AM	01:00				
11:00AM	11:00		6:15PM	18:15		1:15AM	01:15				
11:15AM	11:15		6:30PM	18:30		1:30AM	01:30				
11:30AM	11:30		6:45PM	18:45		1:45AM	01:45				
11:45AM	11:45		7:00PM	19:00		2:00AM	02:00				
12:00PM	12:00		7:15PM	19:15		2:15AM	02:15				
12:15PM	12:15		7:30PM	19:30		2:45AM	02:45				
12:30PM	12:30		7:45PM	19:45		3:00AM	03:00				
12:45PM	12:45		8:00PM	20:00		3:15AM	03:15				
1:00PM	13:00		8:15PM	20:15		3:30AM	03:30				
1:15PM	13:15		8:30PM	20:30		3:45AM	03:45				
1:30PM	13:30		8:45PM	20:45		4:00AM	04:00				
1:45PM	13:45		9:00PM	21:00		4:15AM	04:15				
2:00PM	14:00		9:15PM	21:15		4:30AM	04:30				
2:15PM	14:15		9:30PM	21:30		4:45AM	04:45				
2:30PM	14:30		9:45PM	21:45		5:00AM	05:00				
2:45PM	14:45		10:00PM	22:00							
3:00PM	15:00										

Date_____   Patient ID_____   Room Number_____

AM MEDS GIVEN? Yes_____

                No_____

PM MEDS GIVEN? Yes_____

                No_____

Results/Progress Notes:

_____

_____

_____

_____

_____

_____

_____

_____

_____

_____

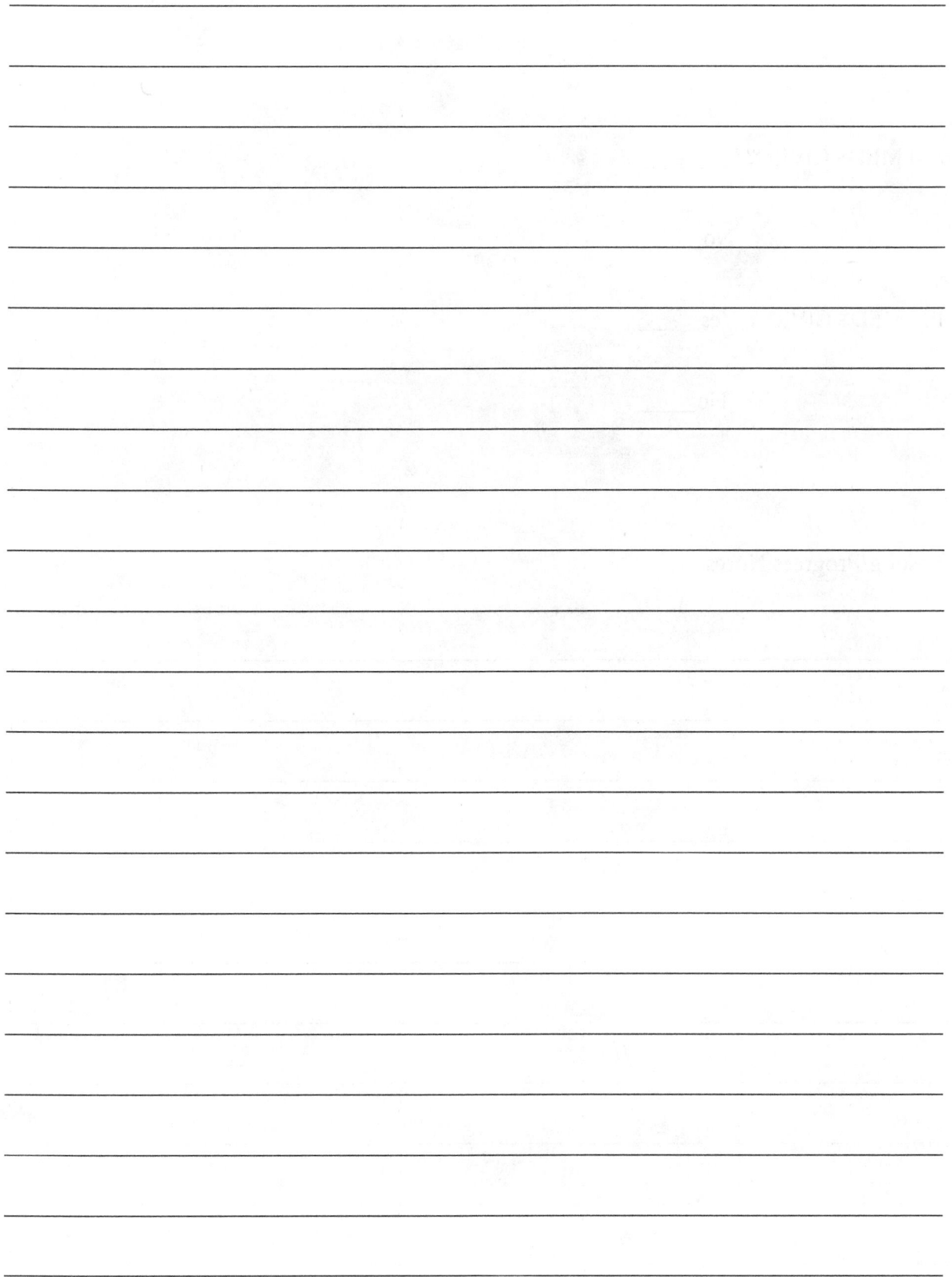

Date_____ Patient ID_____ Room Number_____

Medications   Administering   Mathematical

Instructions   Computations

Medications	Administering Instructions	Mathematical Computations

EST	Military	Notes	EST	Military	Notes	EST	Military	Notes	EST	Military	Notes
8:00 AM	08:00		3:15PM	15:15		10:15PM	22:15		5:15AM	05:15	
8:15 AM	08:15		3:30PM	15:30		10:30PM	22:30		5:30AM	05:30	
8:30AM	08:30		3:45PM	15:45		10:45PM	22:45		5:45AM	05:45	
8:45AM	08:45		4:00PM	16:00		11:00PM	23:00		6:00AM	06:00	
9:00AM	09:00		4:15PM	16:15		11:15PM	23:15		6:15AM	06:15	
9:15AM	09:15		4:30PM	16:30		11:30PM	23:30		6:30AM	06:30	
9:30AM	09:30		4:45PM	16:45		11:45PM	23:45		6:45AM	06:45	
9:45AM	09:45		5:00PM	17:00		12:00AM	24:00		7:00AM	07:00	
10:00AM	10:00		5:15PM	17:15		12:15AM	24:15		7:15AM	07:15	
10:15AM	10:15		5:30PM	17:30		12:30AM	24:30		730AM	07:30	
10:30AM	10:30		5:45PM	17:45		12:45AM	24:45		7:45AM	07:45	
10:45AM	10:45		6:00PM	18:00		1:00AM	01:00				
11:00AM	11:00		6:15PM	18:15		1:15AM	01:15				
11:15AM	11:15		6:30PM	18:30		1:30AM	01:30				
11:30AM	11:30		6:45PM	18:45		1:45AM	01:45				
11:45AM	11:45		7:00PM	19:00		2:00AM	02:00				
12:00PM	12:00		7:15PM	19:15		2:15AM	02:15				
12:15PM	12:15		7:30PM	19:30		2:45AM	02:45				
12:30PM	12:30		7:45PM	19:45		3:00AM	03:00				
12:45PM	12:45		8:00PM	20:00		3:15AM	03:15				
1:00PM	13:00		8:15PM	20:15		3:30AM	03:30				
1:15PM	13:15		8:30PM	20:30		3:45AM	03:45				
1:30PM	13:30		8:45PM	20:45		4:00AM	04:00				
1:45PM	13:45		9:00PM	21:00		4:15AM	04:15				
2:00PM	14:00		9:15PM	21:15		4:30AM	04:30				
2:15PM	14:15		9:30PM	21:30		4:45AM	04:45				
2:30PM	14:30		9:45PM	21:45		5:00AM	05:00				
2:45PM	14:45		10:00PM	22:00							
3:00PM	15:00										

Date_____ Patient ID_____ Room Number_____

AM MEDS GIVEN? Yes_____

No_____

PM MEDS GIVEN? Yes_____

No_____

Results/Progress Notes:

_____

_____

_____

_____

_____

_____

_____

_____

_____

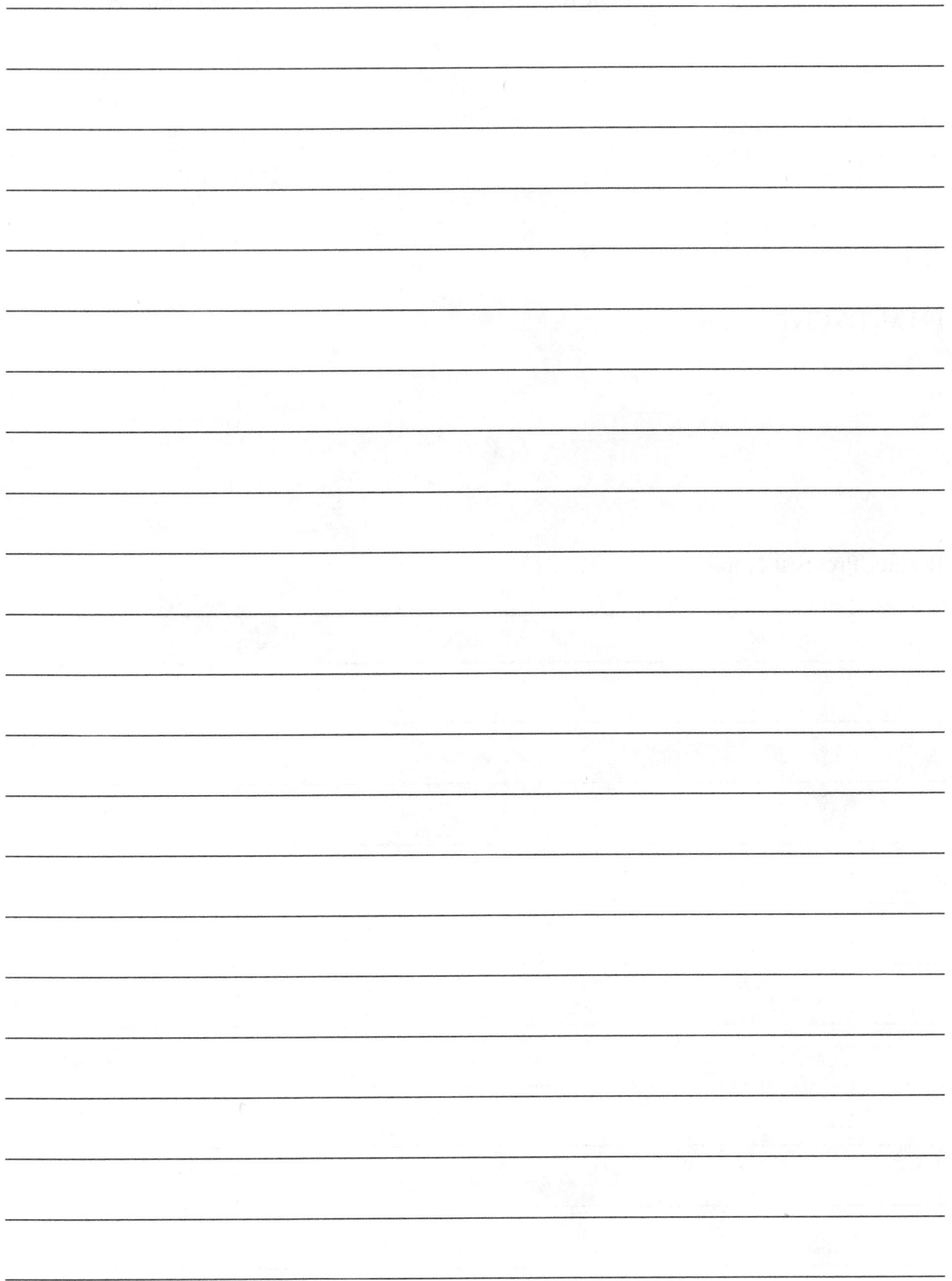

Date_____ Patient ID_____ Room Number_____

Medications	Administering Instructions	Mathematical Computations

EST	Military	Notes	EST	Military	Notes	EST	Military	Notes	EST	Military	Notes
8:00 AM	08:00		3:15PM	15:15		10:15PM	22:15		5:15AM	05:15	
8:15 AM	08:15		3:30PM	15:30		10:30PM	22:30		5:30AM	05:30	
8:30AM	08:30		3:45PM	15:45		10:45PM	22:45		5:45AM	05:45	
8:45AM	08:45		4:00PM	16:00		11:00PM	23:00		6:00AM	06:00	
9:00AM	09:00		4:15PM	16:15		11:15PM	23:15		6:15AM	06:15	
9:15AM	09:15		4:30PM	16:30		11:30PM	23:30		6:30AM	06:30	
9:30AM	09:30		4:45PM	16:45		11:45PM	23:45		6:45AM	06:45	
9:45AM	09:45		5:00PM	17:00		12:00AM	24:00		7:00AM	07:00	
10:00AM	10:00		5:15PM	17:15		12:15AM	24:15		7:15AM	07:15	
10:15AM	10:15		5:30PM	17:30		12:30AM	24:30		730AM	07:30	
10:30AM	10:30		5:45PM	17:45		12:45AM	24:45		7:45AM	07:45	
10:45AM	10:45		6:00PM	18:00		1:00AM	01:00				
11:00AM	11:00		6:15PM	18:15		1:15AM	01:15				
11:15AM	11:15		6:30PM	18:30		1:30AM	01:30				
11:30AM	11:30		6:45PM	18:45		1:45AM	01:45				
11:45AM	11:45		7:00PM	19:00		2:00AM	02:00				
12:00PM	12:00		7:15PM	19:15		2:15AM	02:15				
12:15PM	12:15		7:30PM	19:30		2:45AM	02:45				
12:30PM	12:30		7:45PM	19:45		3:00AM	03:00				
12:45PM	12:45		8:00PM	20:00		3:15AM	03:15				
1:00PM	13:00		8:15PM	20:15		3:30AM	03:30				
1:15PM	13:15		8:30PM	20:30		3:45AM	03:45				
1:30PM	13:30		8:45PM	20:45		4:00AM	04:00				
1:45PM	13:45		9:00PM	21:00		4:15AM	04:15				
2:00PM	14:00		9:15PM	21:15		4:30AM	04:30				
2:15PM	14:15		9:30PM	21:30		4:45AM	04:45				
2:30PM	14:30		9:45PM	21:45		5:00AM	05:00				
2:45PM	14:45		10:00PM	22:00							
3:00PM	15:00										

Date_____ Patient ID_____ Room Number_____

AM MEDS GIVEN? Yes_____

                        No_____

PM MEDS GIVEN? Yes_____

                        No_____

Results/Progress Notes:

_____

_____

_____

_____

_____

_____

_____

_____

_____

_____

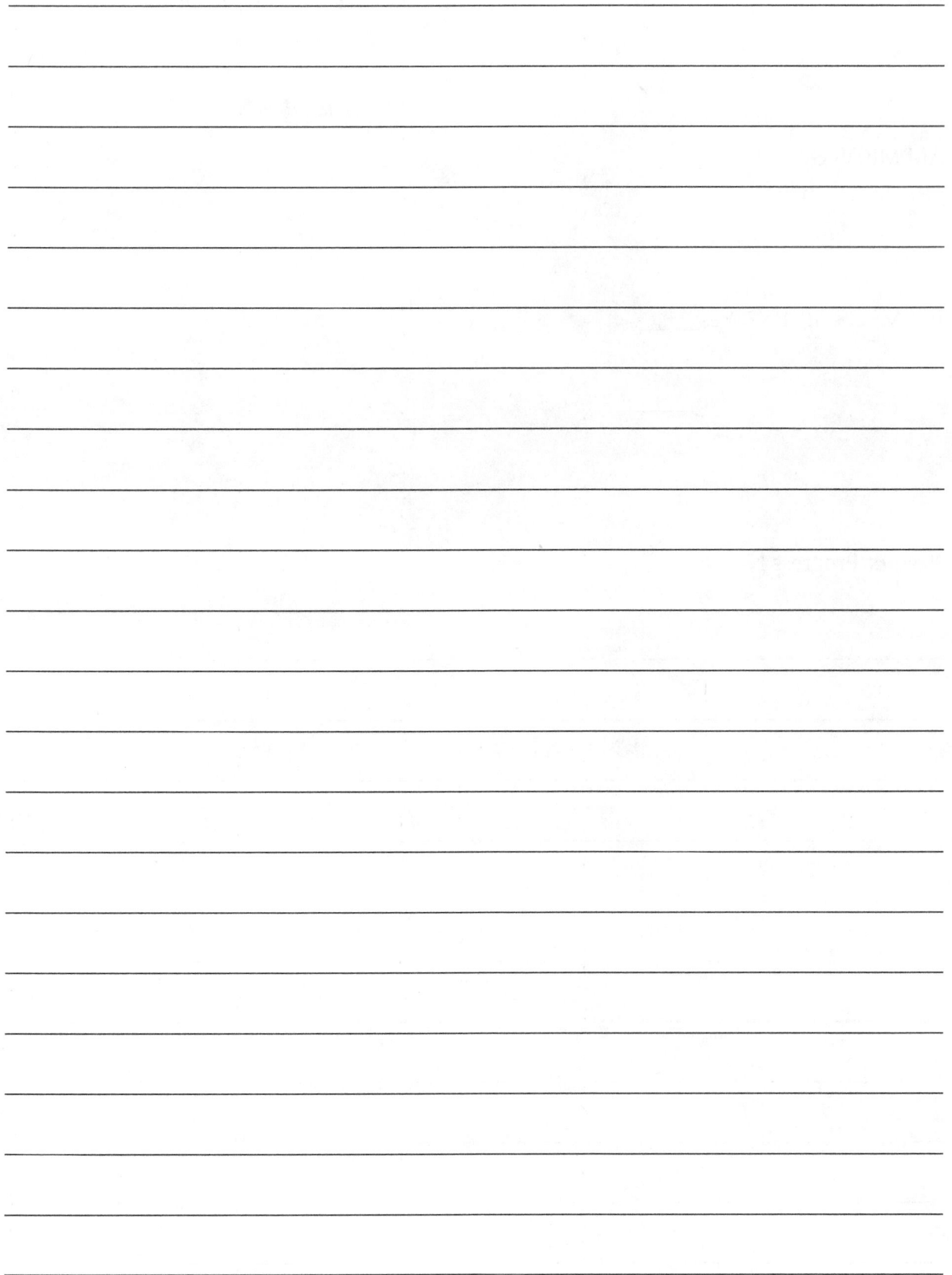

Date_____ Patient ID_____ Room Number_____

Medications

Administering
Instructions

Mathematical
Computations

Medications	Administering Instructions	Mathematical Computations

EST	Military	Notes	EST	Military	Notes	EST	Military	Notes	EST	Military	Notes
8:00 AM	08:00		3:15PM	15:15		10:15PM	22:15		5:15AM	05:15	
8:15 AM	08:15		3:30PM	15:30		10:30PM	22:30		5:30AM	05:30	
8:30AM	08:30		3:45PM	15:45		10:45PM	22:45		5:45AM	05:45	
8:45AM	08:45		4:00PM	16:00		11:00PM	23:00		6:00AM	06:00	
9:00AM	09:00		4:15PM	16:15		11:15PM	23:15		6:15AM	06:15	
9:15AM	09:15		4:30PM	16:30		11:30PM	23:30		6:30AM	06:30	
9:30AM	09:30		4:45PM	16:45		11:45PM	23:45		6:45AM	06:45	
9:45AM	09:45		5:00PM	17:00		12:00AM	24:00		7:00AM	07:00	
10:00AM	10:00		5:15PM	17:15		12:15AM	24:15		7:15AM	07:15	
10:15AM	10:15		5:30PM	17:30		12:30AM	24:30		730AM	07:30	
10:30AM	10:30		5:45PM	17:45		12:45AM	24:45		7:45AM	07:45	
10:45AM	10:45		6:00PM	18:00		1:00AM	01:00				
11:00AM	11:00		6:15PM	18:15		1:15AM	01:15				
11:15AM	11:15		6:30PM	18:30		1:30AM	01:30				
11:30AM	11:30		6:45PM	18:45		1:45AM	01:45				
11:45AM	11:45		7:00PM	19:00		2:00AM	02:00				
12:00PM	12:00		7:15PM	19:15		2:15AM	02:15				
12:15PM	12:15		7:30PM	19:30		2:45AM	02:45				
12:30PM	12:30		7:45PM	19:45		3:00AM	03:00				
12:45PM	12:45		8:00PM	20:00		3:15AM	03:15				
1:00PM	13:00		8:15PM	20:15		3:30AM	03:30				
1:15PM	13:15		8:30PM	20:30		3:45AM	03:45				
1:30PM	13:30		8:45PM	20:45		4:00AM	04:00				
1:45PM	13:45		9:00PM	21:00		4:15AM	04:15				
2:00PM	14:00		9:15PM	21:15		4:30AM	04:30				
2:15PM	14:15		9:30PM	21:30		4:45AM	04:45				
2:30PM	14:30		9:45PM	21:45		5:00AM	05:00				
2:45PM	14:45		10:00PM	22:00							
3:00PM	15:00										

Date_____   Patient ID_____   Room Number_____

AM MEDS GIVEN? Yes_____

          No_____

PM MEDS GIVEN? Yes_____

          No_____

Results/Progress Notes:

_____

_____

_____

_____

_____

_____

_____

_____

_____

_____

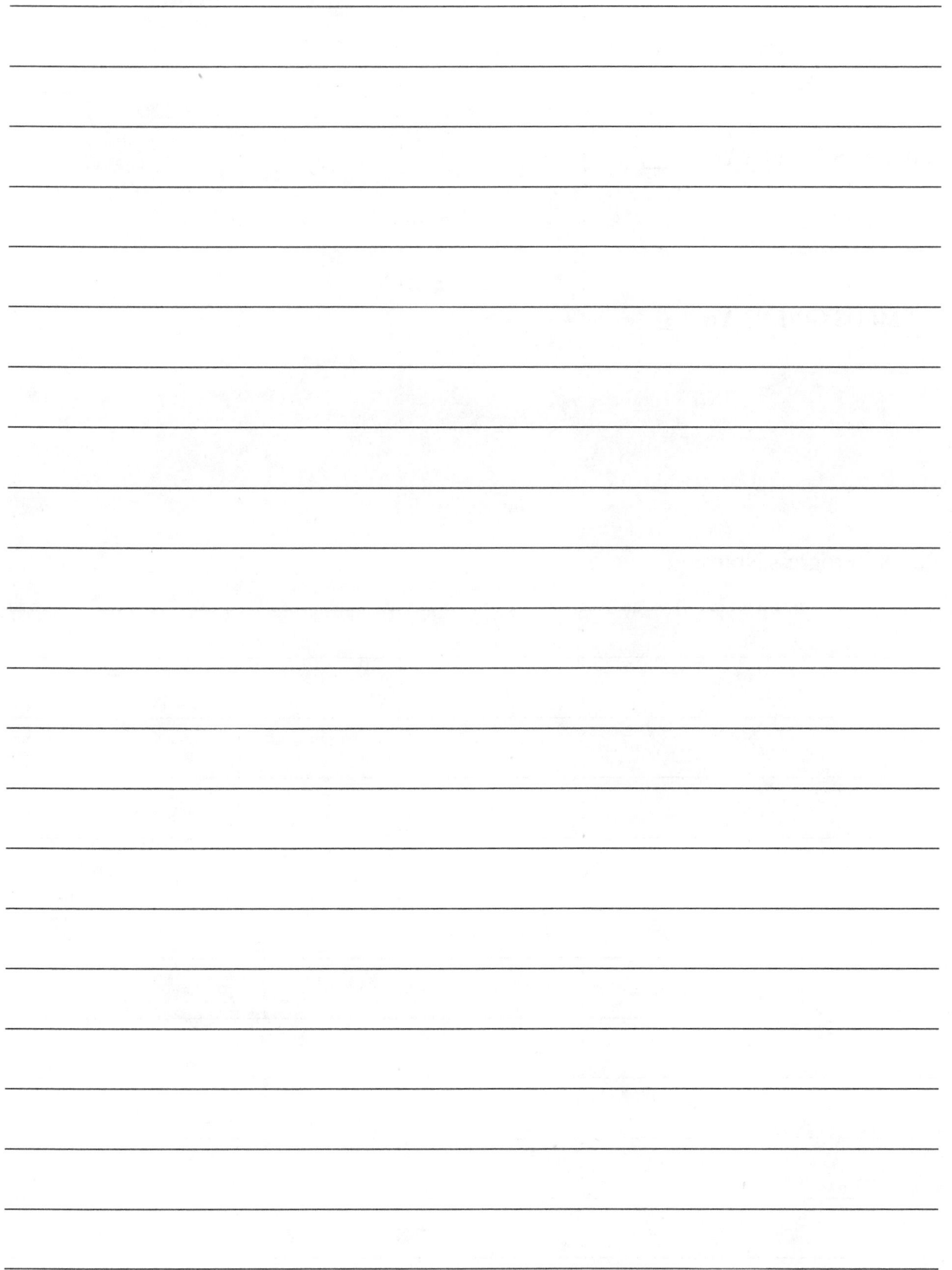

Date_____ Patient ID_____ Room Number_____

	Mathematical
Medications	**Administering**
	Instructions

Mathematical

Computations

Medications	Administering Instructions	Mathematical Computations

EST	Military	Notes	EST	Military	Notes	EST	Military	Notes	EST	Military	Notes
8:00 AM	08:00		3:15PM	15:15		10:15PM	22:15		5:15AM	05:15	
8:15 AM	08:15		3:30PM	15:30		10:30PM	22:30		5:30AM	05:30	
8:30AM	08:30		3:45PM	15:45		10:45PM	22:45		5:45AM	05:45	
8:45AM	08:45		4:00PM	16:00		11:00PM	23:00		6:00AM	06:00	
9:00AM	09:00		4:15PM	16:15		11:15PM	23:15		6:15AM	06:15	
9:15AM	09:15		4:30PM	16:30		11:30PM	23:30		6:30AM	06:30	
9:30AM	09:30		4:45PM	16:45		11:45PM	23:45		6:45AM	06:45	
9:45AM	09:45		5:00PM	17:00		12:00AM	24:00		7:00AM	07:00	
10:00AM	10:00		5:15PM	17:15		12:15AM	24:15		7:15AM	07:15	
10:15AM	10:15		5:30PM	17:30		12:30AM	24:30		730AM	07:30	
10:30AM	10:30		5:45PM	17:45		12:45AM	24:45		7:45AM	07:45	
10:45AM	10:45		6:00PM	18:00		1:00AM	01:00				
11:00AM	11:00		6:15PM	18:15		1:15AM	01:15				
11:15AM	11:15		6:30PM	18:30		1:30AM	01:30				
11:30AM	11:30		6:45PM	18:45		1:45AM	01:45				
11:45AM	11:45		7:00PM	19:00		2:00AM	02:00				
12:00PM	12:00		7:15PM	19:15		2:15AM	02:15				
12:15PM	12:15		7:30PM	19:30		2:45AM	02:45				
12:30PM	12:30		7:45PM	19:45		3:00AM	03:00				
12:45PM	12:45		8:00PM	20:00		3:15AM	03:15				
1:00PM	13:00		8:15PM	20:15		3:30AM	03:30				
1:15PM	13:15		8:30PM	20:30		3:45AM	03:45				
1:30PM	13:30		8:45PM	20:45		4:00AM	04:00				
1:45PM	13:45		9:00PM	21:00		4:15AM	04:15				
2:00PM	14:00		9:15PM	21:15		4:30AM	04:30				
2:15PM	14:15		9:30PM	21:30		4:45AM	04:45				
2:30PM	14:30		9:45PM	21:45		5:00AM	05:00				
2:45PM	14:45		10:00PM	22:00							
3:00PM	15:00										

Date_____ Patient ID_____ Room Number_____

AM MEDS GIVEN? Yes_____

No_____

PM MEDS GIVEN? Yes_____

No_____

Results/Progress Notes:

_____

_____

_____

_____

_____

_____

_____

_____

_____

_____

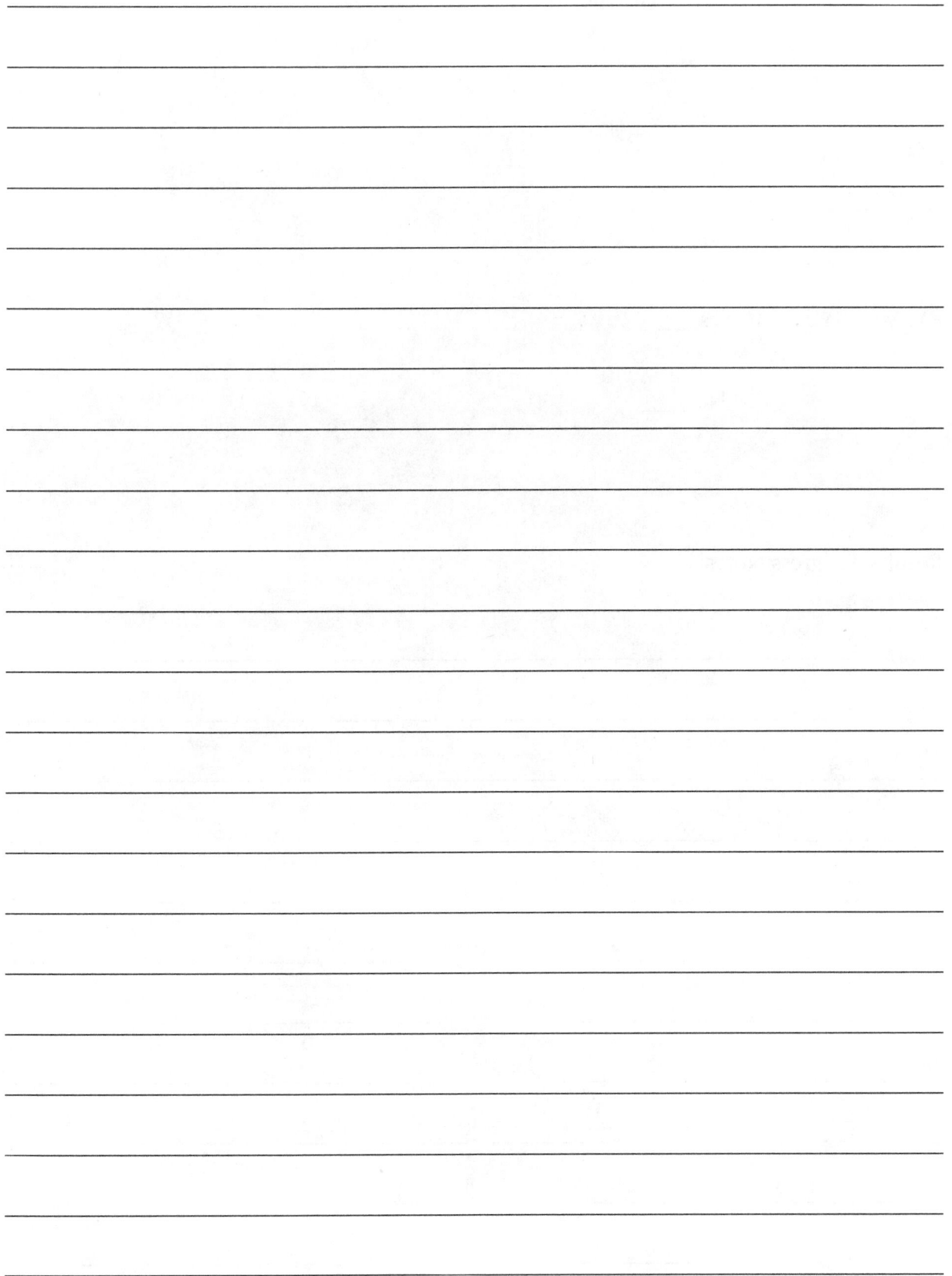

Date_____ Patient ID_____ Room Number_____

Medications	Administering Instructions	Mathematical Computations

EST	Military	Notes	EST	Military	Notes	EST	Military	Notes	EST	Military	Notes
8:00 AM	08:00		3:15PM	15:15		10:15PM	22:15		5:15AM	05:15	
8:15 AM	08:15		3:30PM	15:30		10:30PM	22:30		5:30AM	05:30	
8:30AM	08:30		3:45PM	15:45		10:45PM	22:45		5:45AM	05:45	
8:45AM	08:45		4:00PM	16:00		11:00PM	23:00		6:00AM	06:00	
9:00AM	09:00		4:15PM	16:15		11:15PM	23:15		6:15AM	06:15	
9:15AM	09:15		4:30PM	16:30		11:30PM	23:30		6:30AM	06:30	
9:30AM	09:30		4:45PM	16:45		11:45PM	23:45		6:45AM	06:45	
9:45AM	09:45		5:00PM	17:00		12:00AM	24:00		7:00AM	07:00	
10:00AM	10:00		5:15PM	17:15		12:15AM	24:15		7:15AM	07:15	
10:15AM	10:15		5:30PM	17:30		12:30AM	24:30		730AM	07:30	
10:30AM	10:30		5:45PM	17:45		12:45AM	24:45		7:45AM	07:45	
10:45AM	10:45		6:00PM	18:00		1:00AM	01:00				
11:00AM	11:00		6:15PM	18:15		1:15AM	01:15				
11:15AM	11:15		6:30PM	18:30		1:30AM	01:30				
11:30AM	11:30		6:45PM	18:45		1:45AM	01:45				
11:45AM	11:45		7:00PM	19:00		2:00AM	02:00				
12:00PM	12:00		7:15PM	19:15		2:15AM	02:15				
12:15PM	12:15		7:30PM	19:30		2:45AM	02:45				
12:30PM	12:30		7:45PM	19:45		3:00AM	03:00				
12:45PM	12:45		8:00PM	20:00		3:15AM	03:15				
1:00PM	13:00		8:15PM	20:15		3:30AM	03:30				
1:15PM	13:15		8:30PM	20:30		3:45AM	03:45				
1:30PM	13:30		8:45PM	20:45		4:00AM	04:00				
1:45PM	13:45		9:00PM	21:00		4:15AM	04:15				
2:00PM	14:00		9:15PM	21:15		4:30AM	04:30				
2:15PM	14:15		9:30PM	21:30		4:45AM	04:45				
2:30PM	14:30		9:45PM	21:45		5:00AM	05:00				
2:45PM	14:45		10:00PM	22:00							
3:00PM	15:00										

Date_____ Patient ID_____ Room Number_____

AM MEDS GIVEN? Yes_____

            No_____

PM MEDS GIVEN? Yes_____

            No_____

Results/Progress Notes:

_____

_____

_____

_____

_____

_____

_____

_____

_____

_____

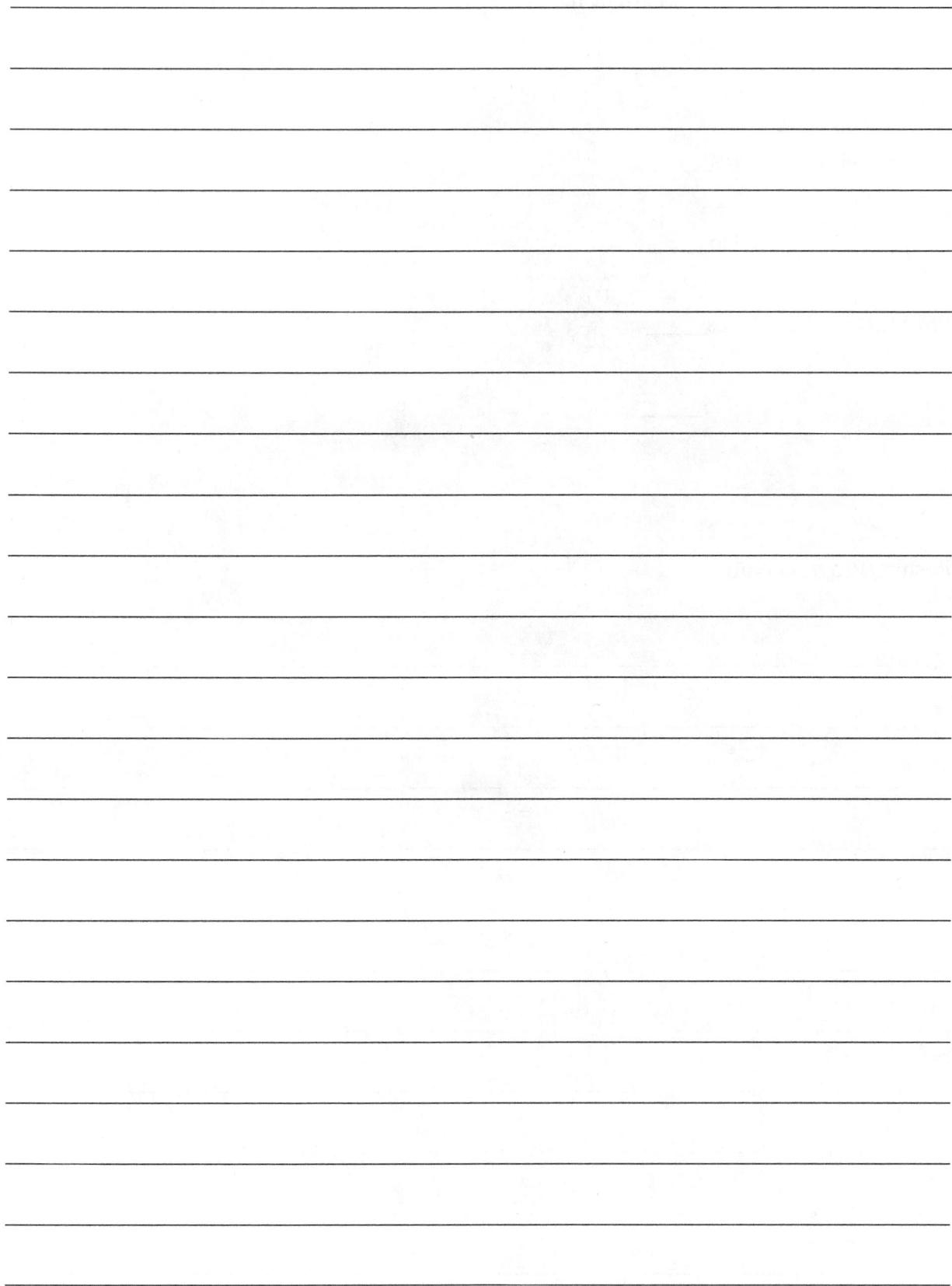

Date_____   Patient ID_____   Room Number_____

| Medications | Administering | Mathematical |
| | Instructions | Computations |

EST	Military	Notes	EST	Military	Notes	EST	Military	Notes	EST	Military	Notes
8:00 AM	08:00		3:15PM	15:15		10:15PM	22:15		5:15AM	05:15	
8:15 AM	08:15		3:30PM	15:30		10:30PM	22:30		5:30AM	05:30	
8:30AM	08:30		3:45PM	15:45		10:45PM	22:45		5:45AM	05:45	
8:45AM	08:45		4:00PM	16:00		11:00PM	23:00		6:00AM	06:00	
9:00AM	09:00		4:15PM	16:15		11:15PM	23:15		6:15AM	06:15	
9:15AM	09:15		4:30PM	16:30		11:30PM	23:30		6:30AM	06:30	
9:30AM	09:30		4:45PM	16:45		11:45PM	23:45		6:45AM	06:45	
9:45AM	09:45		5:00PM	17:00		12:00AM	24:00		7:00AM	07:00	
10:00AM	10:00		5:15PM	17:15		12:15AM	24:15		7:15AM	07:15	
10:15AM	10:15		5:30PM	17:30		12:30AM	24:30		730AM	07:30	
10:30AM	10:30		5:45PM	17:45		12:45AM	24:45		7:45AM	07:45	
10:45AM	10:45		6:00PM	18:00		1:00AM	01:00				
11:00AM	11:00		6:15PM	18:15		1:15AM	01:15				
11:15AM	11:15		6:30PM	18:30		1:30AM	01:30				
11:30AM	11:30		6:45PM	18:45		1:45AM	01:45				
11:45AM	11:45		7:00PM	19:00		2:00AM	02:00				
12:00PM	12:00		7:15PM	19:15		2:15AM	02:15				
12:15PM	12:15		7:30PM	19:30		2:45AM	02:45				
12:30PM	12:30		7:45PM	19:45		3:00AM	03:00				
12:45PM	12:45		8:00PM	20:00		3:15AM	03:15				
1:00PM	13:00		8:15PM	20:15		3:30AM	03:30				
1:15PM	13:15		8:30PM	20:30		3:45AM	03:45				
1:30PM	13:30		8:45PM	20:45		4:00AM	04:00				
1:45PM	13:45		9:00PM	21:00		4:15AM	04:15				
2:00PM	14:00		9:15PM	21:15		4:30AM	04:30				
2:15PM	14:15		9:30PM	21:30		4:45AM	04:45				
2:30PM	14:30		9:45PM	21:45		5:00AM	05:00				
2:45PM	14:45		10:00PM	22:00							
3:00PM	15:00										

Date_____   Patient ID_____   Room Number_____

AM MEDS GIVEN? Yes_____

                     No_____

PM MEDS GIVEN? Yes_____

                     No_____

Results/Progress Notes:

_____

_____

_____

_____

_____

_____

_____

_____

_____

_____

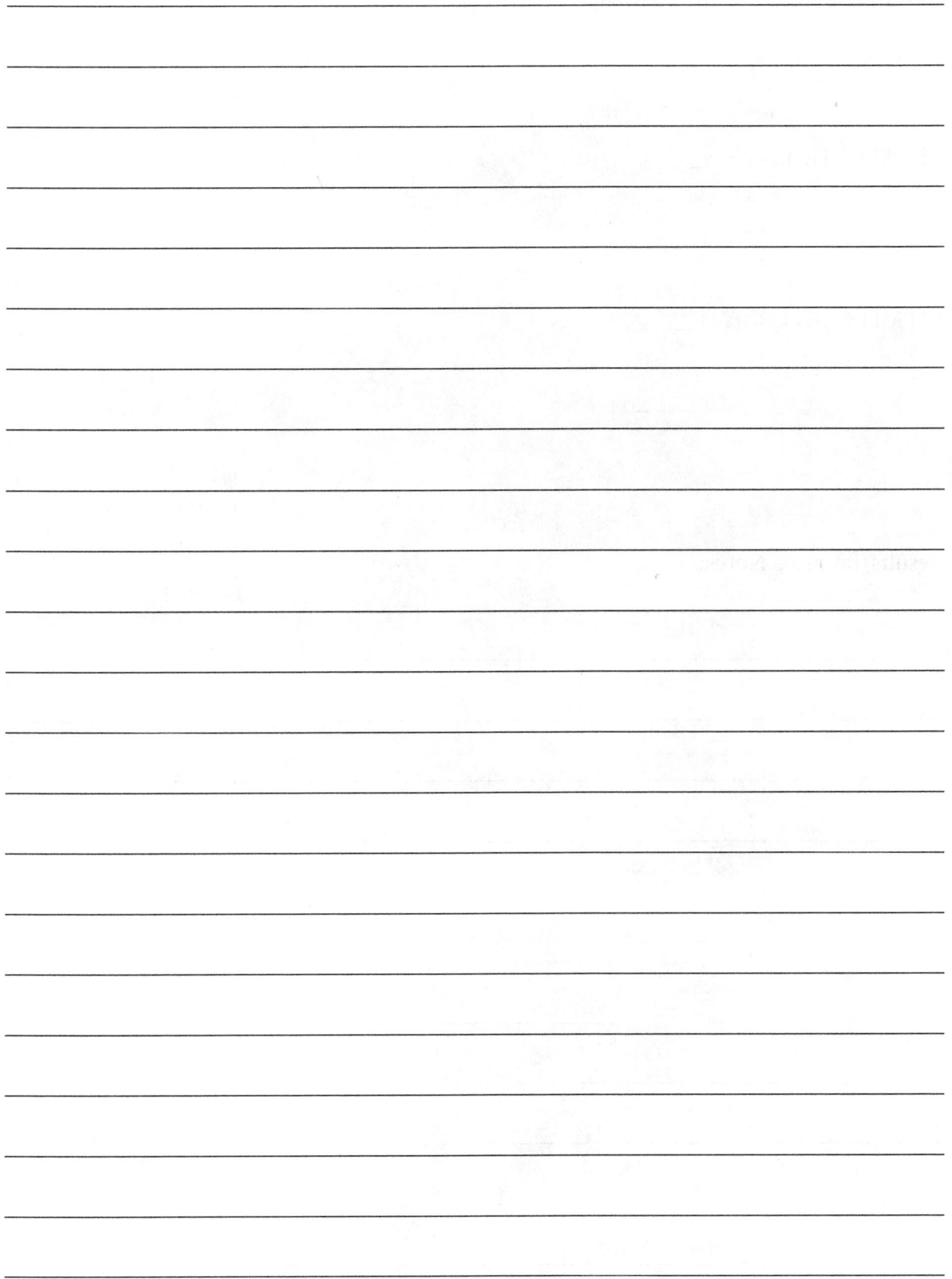

Date_____ Patient ID_____ Room Number_____

Medications	Administering Instructions

Mathematical Computations

EST	Military	Notes	EST	Military	Notes	EST	Military	Notes	EST	Military	Notes
8:00 AM	08:00		3:15PM	15:15		10:15PM	22:15		5:15AM	05:15	
8:15 AM	08:15		3:30PM	15:30		10:30PM	22:30		5:30AM	05:30	
8:30AM	08:30		3:45PM	15:45		10:45PM	22:45		5:45AM	05:45	
8:45AM	08:45		4:00PM	16:00		11:00PM	23:00		6:00AM	06:00	
9:00AM	09:00		4:15PM	16:15		11:15PM	23:15		6:15AM	06:15	
9:15AM	09:15		4:30PM	16:30		11:30PM	23:30		6:30AM	06:30	
9:30AM	09:30		4:45PM	16:45		11:45PM	23:45		6:45AM	06:45	
9:45AM	09:45		5:00PM	17:00		12:00AM	24:00		7:00AM	07:00	
10:00AM	10:00		5:15PM	17:15		12:15AM	24:15		7:15AM	07:15	
10:15AM	10:15		5:30PM	17:30		12:30AM	24:30		730AM	07:30	
10:30AM	10:30		5:45PM	17:45		12:45AM	24:45		7:45AM	07:45	
10:45AM	10:45		6:00PM	18:00		1:00AM	01:00				
11:00AM	11:00		6:15PM	18:15		1:15AM	01:15				
11:15AM	11:15		6:30PM	18:30		1:30AM	01:30				
11:30AM	11:30		6:45PM	18:45		1:45AM	01:45				
11:45AM	11:45		7:00PM	19:00		2:00AM	02:00				
12:00PM	12:00		7:15PM	19:15		2:15AM	02:15				
12:15PM	12:15		7:30PM	19:30		2:45AM	02:45				
12:30PM	12:30		7:45PM	19:45		3:00AM	03:00				
12:45PM	12:45		8:00PM	20:00		3:15AM	03:15				
1:00PM	13:00		8:15PM	20:15		3:30AM	03:30				
1:15PM	13:15		8:30PM	20:30		3:45AM	03:45				
1:30PM	13:30		8:45PM	20:45		4:00AM	04:00				
1:45PM	13:45		9:00PM	21:00		4:15AM	04:15				
2:00PM	14:00		9:15PM	21:15		4:30AM	04:30				
2:15PM	14:15		9:30PM	21:30		4:45AM	04:45				
2:30PM	14:30		9:45PM	21:45		5:00AM	05:00				
2:45PM	14:45		10:00PM	22:00							
3:00PM	15:00										

Date_____   Patient ID_____   Room Number_____

AM MEDS GIVEN? Yes_____

              No_____

PM MEDS GIVEN? Yes_____

              No_____

Results/Progress Notes:

_____

_____

_____

_____

_____

_____

_____

_____

_____

_____

_____

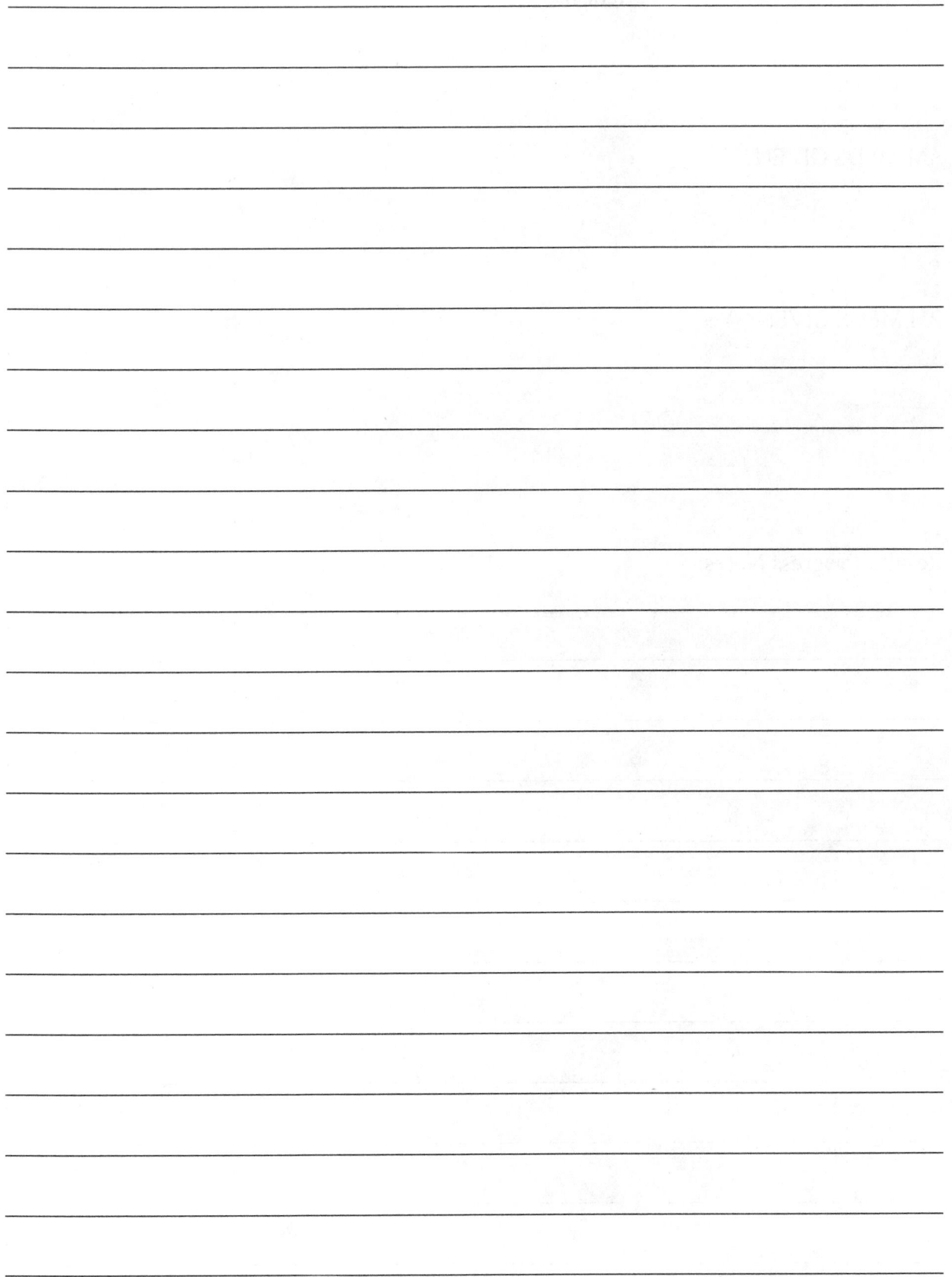

Date_____ Patient ID_____ Room Number_____

Medications	Administering Instructions	Mathematical Computations

EST	Military	Notes	EST	Military	Notes	EST	Military	Notes	EST	Military	Notes
8:00 AM	08:00		3:15PM	15:15		10:15PM	22:15		5:15AM	05:15	
8:15 AM	08:15		3:30PM	15:30		10:30PM	22:30		5:30AM	05:30	
8:30AM	08:30		3:45PM	15:45		10:45PM	22:45		5:45AM	05:45	
8:45AM	08:45		4:00PM	16:00		11:00PM	23:00		6:00AM	06:00	
9:00AM	09:00		4:15PM	16:15		11:15PM	23:15		6:15AM	06:15	
9:15AM	09:15		4:30PM	16:30		11:30PM	23:30		6:30AM	06:30	
9:30AM	09:30		4:45PM	16:45		11:45PM	23:45		6:45AM	06:45	
9:45AM	09:45		5:00PM	17:00		12:00AM	24:00		7:00AM	07:00	
10:00AM	10:00		5:15PM	17:15		12:15AM	24:15		7:15AM	07:15	
10:15AM	10:15		5:30PM	17:30		12:30AM	24:30		730AM	07:30	
10:30AM	10:30		5:45PM	17:45		12:45AM	24:45		7:45AM	07:45	
10:45AM	10:45		6:00PM	18:00		1:00AM	01:00				
11:00AM	11:00		6:15PM	18:15		1:15AM	01:15				
11:15AM	11:15		6:30PM	18:30		1:30AM	01:30				
11:30AM	11:30		6:45PM	18:45		1:45AM	01:45				
11:45AM	11:45		7:00PM	19:00		2:00AM	02:00				
12:00PM	12:00		7:15PM	19:15		2:15AM	02:15				
12:15PM	12:15		7:30PM	19:30		2:45AM	02:45				
12:30PM	12:30		7:45PM	19:45		3:00AM	03:00				
12:45PM	12:45		8:00PM	20:00		3:15AM	03:15				
1:00PM	13:00		8:15PM	20:15		3:30AM	03:30				
1:15PM	13:15		8:30PM	20:30		3:45AM	03:45				
1:30PM	13:30		8:45PM	20:45		4:00AM	04:00				
1:45PM	13:45		9:00PM	21:00		4:15AM	04:15				
2:00PM	14:00		9:15PM	21:15		4:30AM	04:30				
2:15PM	14:15		9:30PM	21:30		4:45AM	04:45				
2:30PM	14:30		9:45PM	21:45		5:00AM	05:00				
2:45PM	14:45		10:00PM	22:00							
3:00PM	15:00										

Date_____   Patient ID_____   Room Number_____

AM MEDS GIVEN? Yes_____

                No_____

PM MEDS GIVEN? Yes_____

                No_____

Results/Progress Notes:

_____

_____

_____

_____

_____

_____

_____

_____

_____

_____

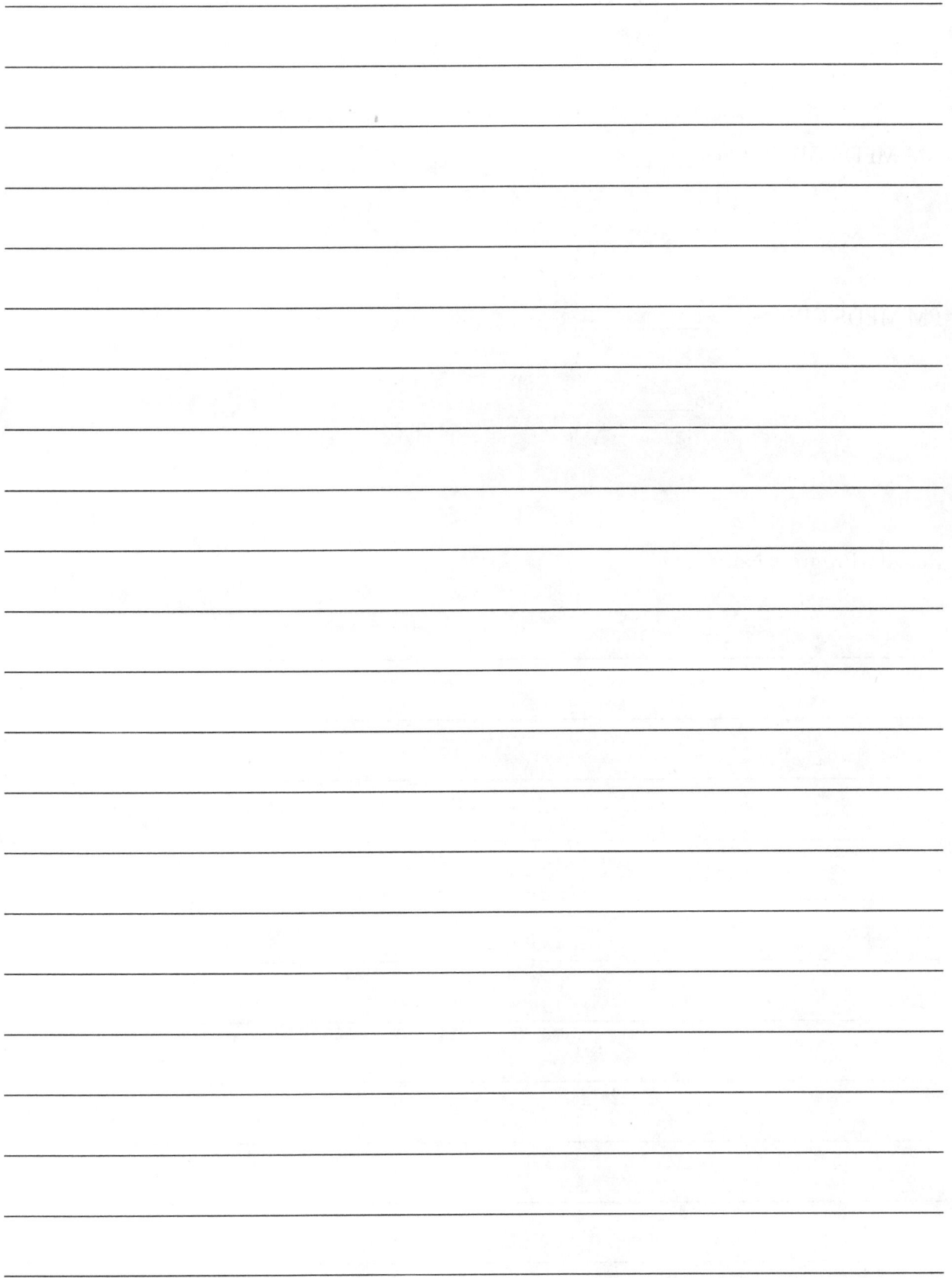

Date_____ Patient ID_____ Room Number_____

Medications   Administering   Mathematical

                     Instructions   Computations

EST	Military	Notes	EST	Military	Notes	EST	Military	Notes	EST	Military	Notes
8:00 AM	08:00		3:15PM	15:15		10:15PM	22:15		5:15AM	05:15	
8:15 AM	08:15		3:30PM	15:30		10:30PM	22:30		5:30AM	05:30	
8:30AM	08:30		3:45PM	15:45		10:45PM	22:45		5:45AM	05:45	
8:45AM	08:45		4:00PM	16:00		11:00PM	23:00		6:00AM	06:00	
9:00AM	09:00		4:15PM	16:15		11:15PM	23:15		6:15AM	06:15	
9:15AM	09:15		4:30PM	16:30		11:30PM	23:30		6:30AM	06:30	
9:30AM	09:30		4:45PM	16:45		11:45PM	23:45		6:45AM	06:45	
9:45AM	09:45		5:00PM	17:00		12:00AM	24:00		7:00AM	07:00	
10:00AM	10:00		5:15PM	17:15		12:15AM	24:15		7:15AM	07:15	
10:15AM	10:15		5:30PM	17:30		12:30AM	24:30		730AM	07:30	
10:30AM	10:30		5:45PM	17:45		12:45AM	24:45		7:45AM	07:45	
10:45AM	10:45		6:00PM	18:00		1:00AM	01:00				
11:00AM	11:00		6:15PM	18:15		1:15AM	01:15				
11:15AM	11:15		6:30PM	18:30		1:30AM	01:30				
11:30AM	11:30		6:45PM	18:45		1:45AM	01:45				
11:45AM	11:45		7:00PM	19:00		2:00AM	02:00				
12:00PM	12:00		7:15PM	19:15		2:15AM	02:15				
12:15PM	12:15		7:30PM	19:30		2:45AM	02:45				
12:30PM	12:30		7:45PM	19:45		3:00AM	03:00				
12:45PM	12:45		8:00PM	20:00		3:15AM	03:15				
1:00PM	13:00		8:15PM	20:15		3:30AM	03:30				
1:15PM	13:15		8:30PM	20:30		3:45AM	03:45				
1:30PM	13:30		8:45PM	20:45		4:00AM	04:00				
1:45PM	13:45		9:00PM	21:00		4:15AM	04:15				
2:00PM	14:00		9:15PM	21:15		4:30AM	04:30				
2:15PM	14:15		9:30PM	21:30		4:45AM	04:45				
2:30PM	14:30		9:45PM	21:45		5:00AM	05:00				
2:45PM	14:45		10:00PM	22:00							
3:00PM	15:00										

Date_____   Patient ID_____   Room Number_____

AM MEDS GIVEN? Yes_____

                 No_____

PM MEDS GIVEN? Yes_____

                 No_____

Results/Progress Notes:

_____

_____

_____

_____

_____

_____

_____

_____

_____

_____

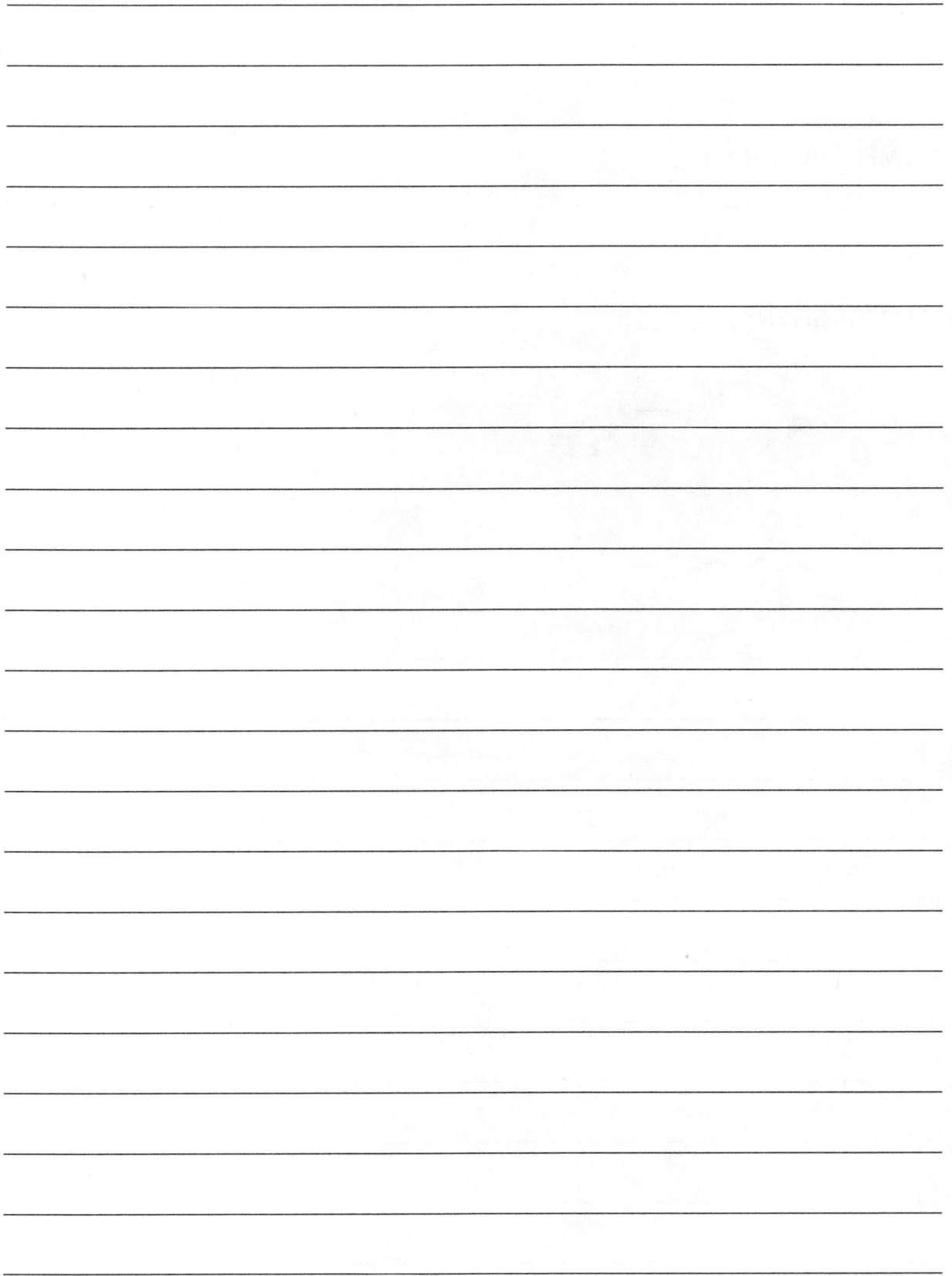

Date_____ Patient ID_____ Room Number_____

Medications	Administering Instructions	Mathematical Computations

EST	Military	Notes	EST	Military	Notes	EST	Military	Notes	EST	Military	Notes
8:00 AM	08:00		3:15PM	15:15		10:15PM	22:15		5:15AM	05:15	
8:15 AM	08:15		3:30PM	15:30		10:30PM	22:30		5:30AM	05:30	
8:30AM	08:30		3:45PM	15:45		10:45PM	22:45		5:45AM	05:45	
8:45AM	08:45		4:00PM	16:00		11:00PM	23:00		6:00AM	06:00	
9:00AM	09:00		4:15PM	16:15		11:15PM	23:15		6:15AM	06:15	
9:15AM	09:15		4:30PM	16:30		11:30PM	23:30		6:30AM	06:30	
9:30AM	09:30		4:45PM	16:45		11:45PM	23:45		6:45AM	06:45	
9:45AM	09:45		5:00PM	17:00		12:00AM	24:00		7:00AM	07:00	
10:00AM	10:00		5:15PM	17:15		12:15AM	24:15		7:15AM	07:15	
10:15AM	10:15		5:30PM	17:30		12:30AM	24:30		730AM	07:30	
10:30AM	10:30		5:45PM	17:45		12:45AM	24:45		7:45AM	07:45	
10:45AM	10:45		6:00PM	18:00		1:00AM	01:00				
11:00AM	11:00		6:15PM	18:15		1:15AM	01:15				
11:15AM	11:15		6:30PM	18:30		1:30AM	01:30				
11:30AM	11:30		6:45PM	18:45		1:45AM	01:45				
11:45AM	11:45		7:00PM	19:00		2:00AM	02:00				
12:00PM	12:00		7:15PM	19:15		2:15AM	02:15				
12:15PM	12:15		7:30PM	19:30		2:45AM	02:45				
12:30PM	12:30		7:45PM	19:45		3:00AM	03:00				
12:45PM	12:45		8:00PM	20:00		3:15AM	03:15				
1:00PM	13:00		8:15PM	20:15		3:30AM	03:30				
1:15PM	13:15		8:30PM	20:30		3:45AM	03:45				
1:30PM	13:30		8:45PM	20:45		4:00AM	04:00				
1:45PM	13:45		9:00PM	21:00		4:15AM	04:15				
2:00PM	14:00		9:15PM	21:15		4:30AM	04:30				
2:15PM	14:15		9:30PM	21:30		4:45AM	04:45				
2:30PM	14:30		9:45PM	21:45		5:00AM	05:00				
2:45PM	14:45		10:00PM	22:00							
3:00PM	15:00										

Date_____ Patient ID_____ Room Number_____

AM MEDS GIVEN? Yes_____

No_____

PM MEDS GIVEN? Yes_____

No_____

Results/Progress Notes:

_____

_____

_____

_____

_____

_____

_____

_____

_____

_____

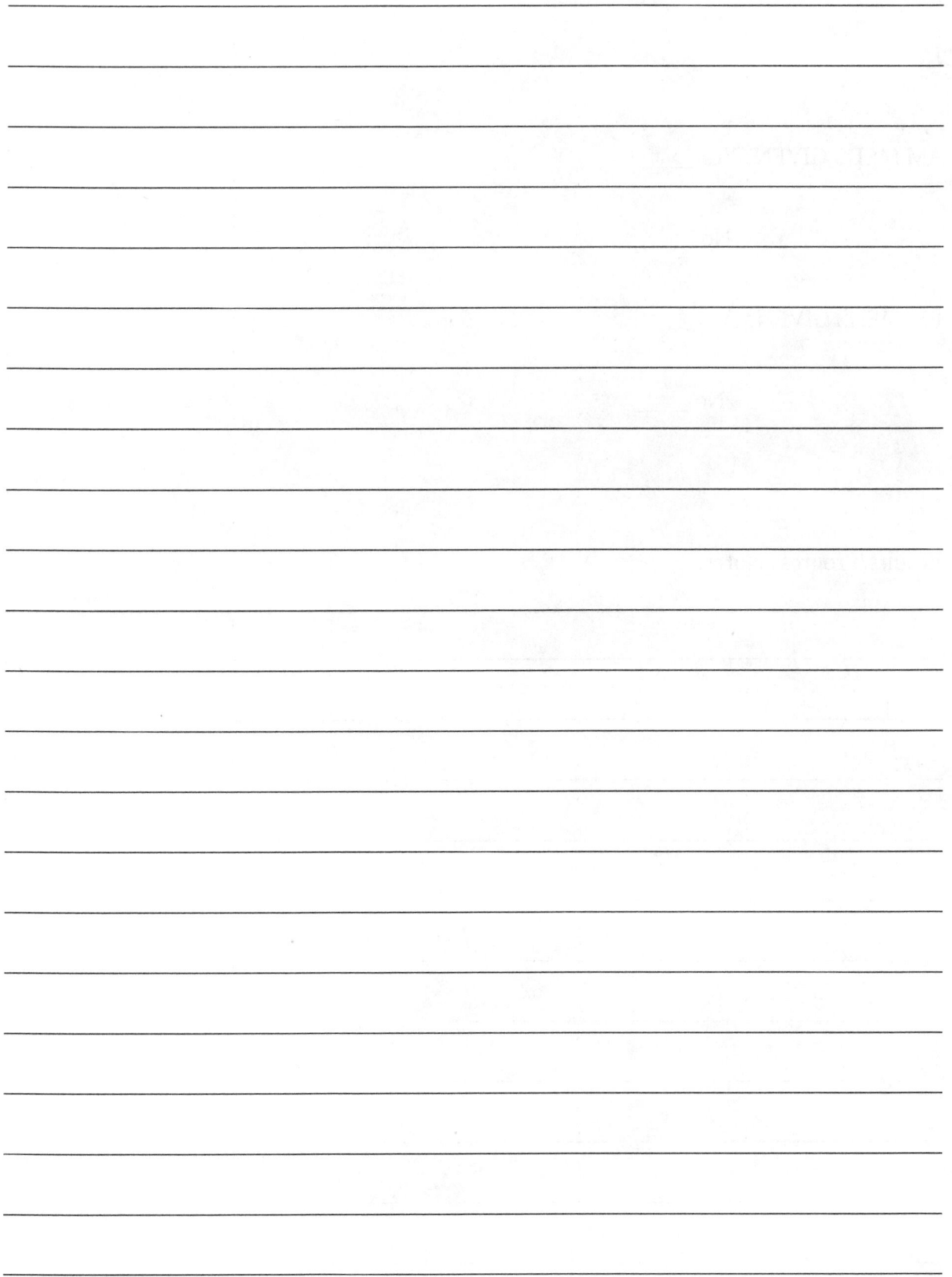

Date_____ Patient ID_____ Room Number_____

Medications	Administering Instructions	Mathematical Computations

EST	Military	Notes	EST	Military	Notes	EST	Military	Notes	EST	Military	Notes
8:00 AM	08:00		3:15PM	15:15		10:15PM	22:15		5:15AM	05:15	
8:15 AM	08:15		3:30PM	15:30		10:30PM	22:30		5:30AM	05:30	
8:30AM	08:30		3:45PM	15:45		10:45PM	22:45		5:45AM	05:45	
8:45AM	08:45		4:00PM	16:00		11:00PM	23:00		6:00AM	06:00	
9:00AM	09:00		4:15PM	16:15		11:15PM	23:15		6:15AM	06:15	
9:15AM	09:15		4:30PM	16:30		11:30PM	23:30		6:30AM	06:30	
9:30AM	09:30		4:45PM	16:45		11:45PM	23:45		6:45AM	06:45	
9:45AM	09:45		5:00PM	17:00		12:00AM	24:00		7:00AM	07:00	
10:00AM	10:00		5:15PM	17:15		12:15AM	24:15		7:15AM	07:15	
10:15AM	10:15		5:30PM	17:30		12:30AM	24:30		730AM	07:30	
10:30AM	10:30		5:45PM	17:45		12:45AM	24:45		7:45AM	07:45	
10:45AM	10:45		6:00PM	18:00		1:00AM	01:00				
11:00AM	11:00		6:15PM	18:15		1:15AM	01:15				
11:15AM	11:15		6:30PM	18:30		1:30AM	01:30				
11:30AM	11:30		6:45PM	18:45		1:45AM	01:45				
11:45AM	11:45		7:00PM	19:00		2:00AM	02:00				
12:00PM	12:00		7:15PM	19:15		2:15AM	02:15				
12:15PM	12:15		7:30PM	19:30		2:45AM	02:45				
12:30PM	12:30		7:45PM	19:45		3:00AM	03:00				
12:45PM	12:45		8:00PM	20:00		3:15AM	03:15				
1:00PM	13:00		8:15PM	20:15		3:30AM	03:30				
1:15PM	13:15		8:30PM	20:30		3:45AM	03:45				
1:30PM	13:30		8:45PM	20:45		4:00AM	04:00				
1:45PM	13:45		9:00PM	21:00		4:15AM	04:15				
2:00PM	14:00		9:15PM	21:15		4:30AM	04:30				
2:15PM	14:15		9:30PM	21:30		4:45AM	04:45				
2:30PM	14:30		9:45PM	21:45		5:00AM	05:00				
2:45PM	14:45		10:00PM	22:00							
3:00PM	15:00										

Date_____ Patient ID_____ Room Number_____

AM MEDS GIVEN? Yes_____

No_____

PM MEDS GIVEN? Yes_____

No_____

Results/Progress Notes:

_____

_____

_____

_____

_____

_____

_____

_____

_____

_____

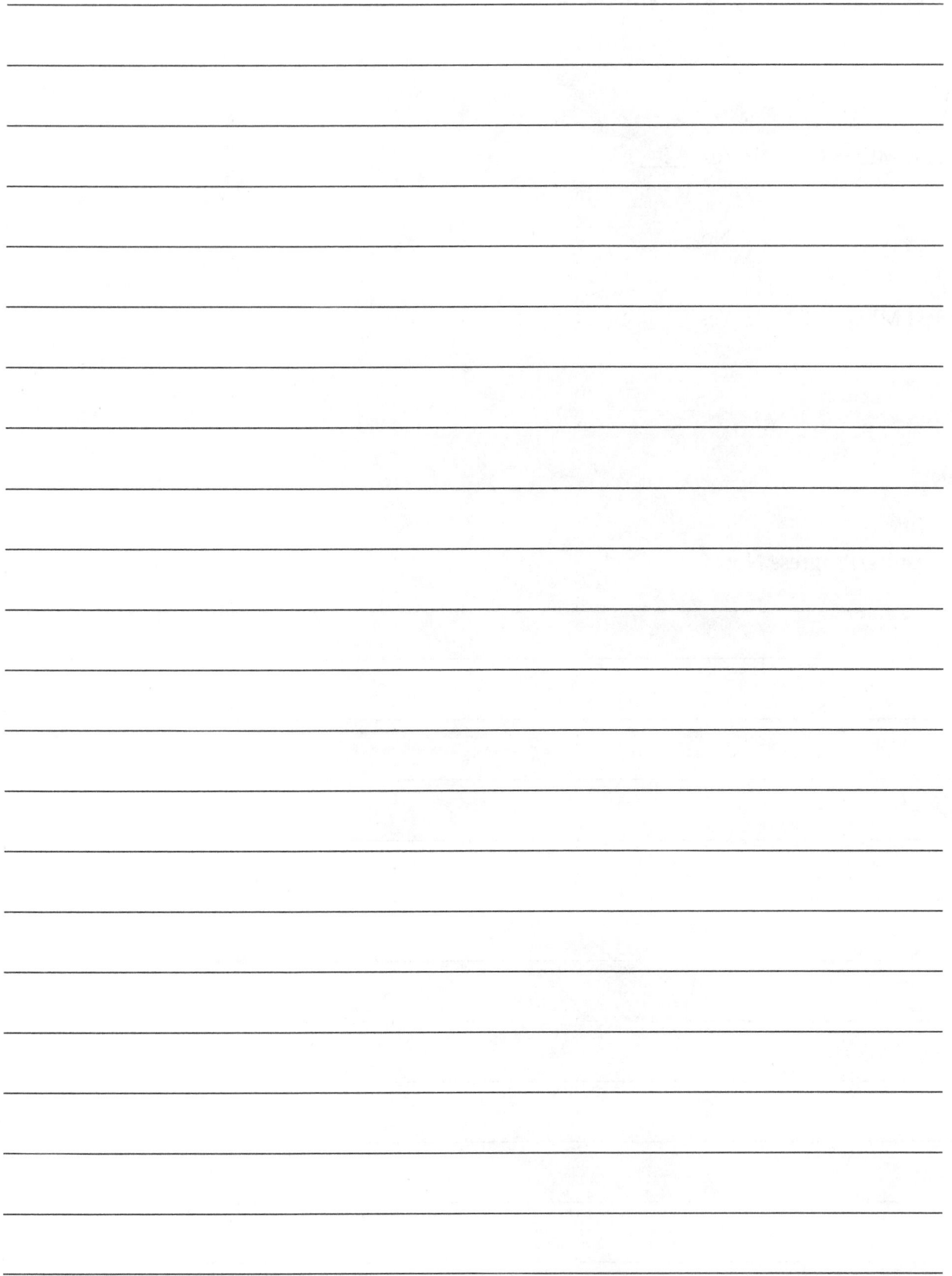

Date_____ Patient ID_____ Room Number_____

Medications	Administering Instructions

Mathematical Computations

EST	Military	Notes	EST	Military	Notes	EST	Military	Notes	EST	Military	Notes
8:00 AM	08:00		3:15PM	15:15		10:15PM	22:15		5:15AM	05:15	
8:15 AM	08:15		3:30PM	15:30		10:30PM	22:30		5:30AM	05:30	
8:30AM	08:30		3:45PM	15:45		10:45PM	22:45		5:45AM	05:45	
8:45AM	08:45		4:00PM	16:00		11:00PM	23:00		6:00AM	06:00	
9:00AM	09:00		4:15PM	16:15		11:15PM	23:15		6:15AM	06:15	
9:15AM	09:15		4:30PM	16:30		11:30PM	23:30		6:30AM	06:30	
9:30AM	09:30		4:45PM	16:45		11:45PM	23:45		6:45AM	06:45	
9:45AM	09:45		5:00PM	17:00		12:00AM	24:00		7:00AM	07:00	
10:00AM	10:00		5:15PM	17:15		12:15AM	24:15		7:15AM	07:15	
10:15AM	10:15		5:30PM	17:30		12:30AM	24:30		730AM	07:30	
10:30AM	10:30		5:45PM	17:45		12:45AM	24:45		7:45AM	07:45	
10:45AM	10:45		6:00PM	18:00		1:00AM	01:00				
11:00AM	11:00		6:15PM	18:15		1:15AM	01:15				
11:15AM	11:15		6:30PM	18:30		1:30AM	01:30				
11:30AM	11:30		6:45PM	18:45		1:45AM	01:45				
11:45AM	11:45		7:00PM	19:00		2:00AM	02:00				
12:00PM	12:00		7:15PM	19:15		2:15AM	02:15				
12:15PM	12:15		7:30PM	19:30		2:45AM	02:45				
12:30PM	12:30		7:45PM	19:45		3:00AM	03:00				
12:45PM	12:45		8:00PM	20:00		3:15AM	03:15				
1:00PM	13:00		8:15PM	20:15		3:30AM	03:30				
1:15PM	13:15		8:30PM	20:30		3:45AM	03:45				
1:30PM	13:30		8:45PM	20:45		4:00AM	04:00				
1:45PM	13:45		9:00PM	21:00		4:15AM	04:15				
2:00PM	14:00		9:15PM	21:15		4:30AM	04:30				
2:15PM	14:15		9:30PM	21:30		4:45AM	04:45				
2:30PM	14:30		9:45PM	21:45		5:00AM	05:00				
2:45PM	14:45		10:00PM	22:00							
3:00PM	15:00										

Date_____ Patient ID_____ Room Number_____

AM MEDS GIVEN? Yes_____

No_____

PM MEDS GIVEN? Yes_____

No_____

Results/Progress Notes:

_____

_____

_____

_____

_____

_____

_____

_____

_____

_____

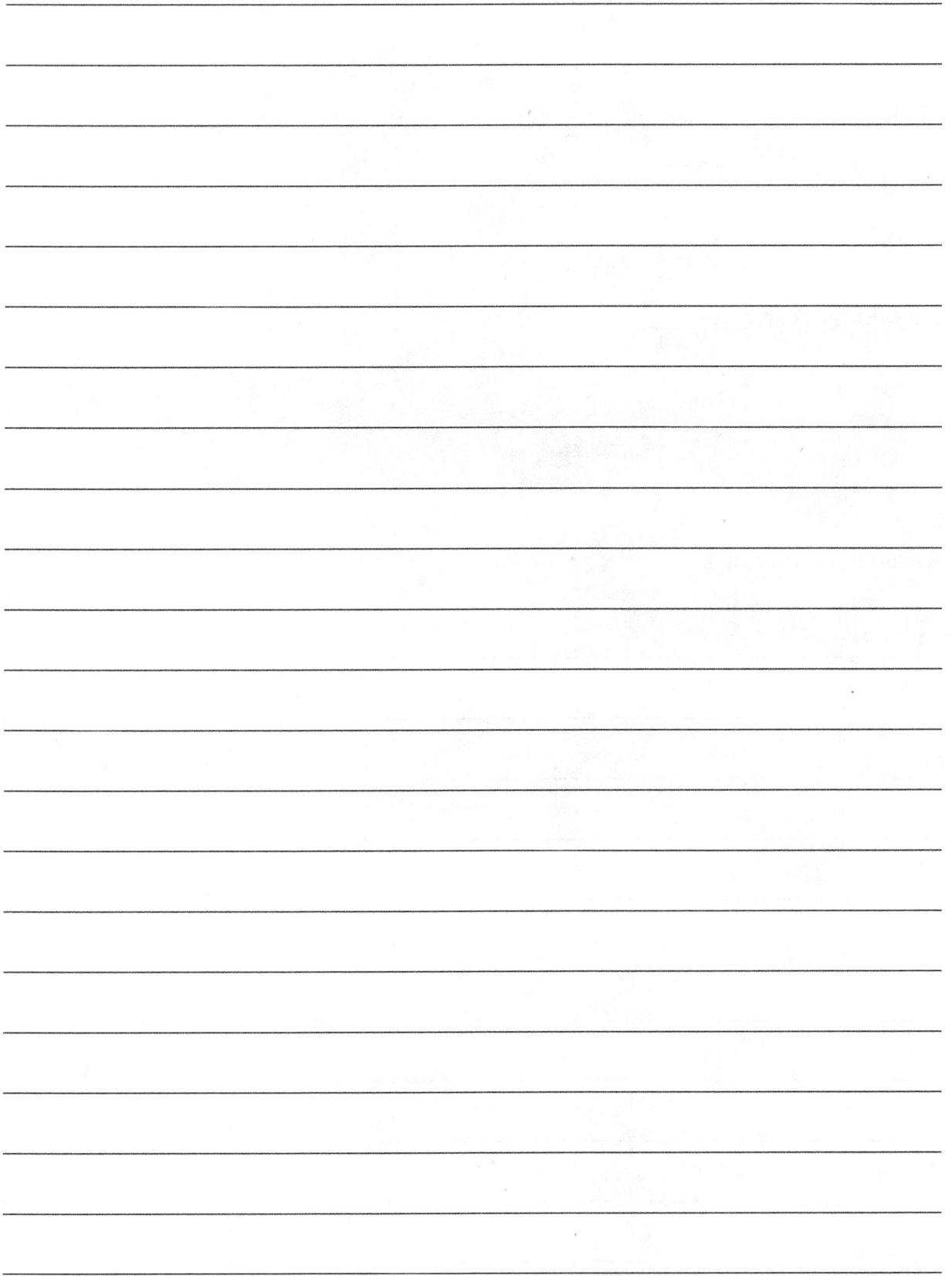

Date_____ Patient ID_____ Room Number_____

Medications	Administering Instructions	Mathematical Computations

EST	Military	Notes	EST	Military	Notes	EST	Military	Notes	EST	Military	Notes
8:00 AM	08:00		3:15PM	15:15		10:15PM	22:15		5:15AM	05:15	
8:15 AM	08:15		3:30PM	15:30		10:30PM	22:30		5:30AM	05:30	
8:30AM	08:30		3:45PM	15:45		10:45PM	22:45		5:45AM	05:45	
8:45AM	08:45		4:00PM	16:00		11:00PM	23:00		6:00AM	06:00	
9:00AM	09:00		4:15PM	16:15		11:15PM	23:15		6:15AM	06:15	
9:15AM	09:15		4:30PM	16:30		11:30PM	23:30		6:30AM	06:30	
9:30AM	09:30		4:45PM	16:45		11:45PM	23:45		6:45AM	06:45	
9:45AM	09:45		5:00PM	17:00		12:00AM	24:00		7:00AM	07:00	
10:00AM	10:00		5:15PM	17:15		12:15AM	24:15		7:15AM	07:15	
10:15AM	10:15		5:30PM	17:30		12:30AM	24:30		730AM	07:30	
10:30AM	10:30		5:45PM	17:45		12:45AM	24:45		7:45AM	07:45	
10:45AM	10:45		6:00PM	18:00		1:00AM	01:00				
11:00AM	11:00		6:15PM	18:15		1:15AM	01:15				
11:15AM	11:15		6:30PM	18:30		1:30AM	01:30				
11:30AM	11:30		6:45PM	18:45		1:45AM	01:45				
11:45AM	11:45		7:00PM	19:00		2:00AM	02:00				
12:00PM	12:00		7:15PM	19:15		2:15AM	02:15				
12:15PM	12:15		7:30PM	19:30		2:45AM	02:45				
12:30PM	12:30		7:45PM	19:45		3:00AM	03:00				
12:45PM	12:45		8:00PM	20:00		3:15AM	03:15				
1:00PM	13:00		8:15PM	20:15		3:30AM	03:30				
1:15PM	13:15		8:30PM	20:30		3:45AM	03:45				
1:30PM	13:30		8:45PM	20:45		4:00AM	04:00				
1:45PM	13:45		9:00PM	21:00		4:15AM	04:15				
2:00PM	14:00		9:15PM	21:15		4:30AM	04:30				
2:15PM	14:15		9:30PM	21:30		4:45AM	04:45				
2:30PM	14:30		9:45PM	21:45		5:00AM	05:00				
2:45PM	14:45		10:00PM	22:00							
3:00PM	15:00										

Date_____ Patient ID_____ Room Number_____

AM MEDS GIVEN? Yes_____

                 No_____

PM MEDS GIVEN? Yes_____

                 No_____

Results/Progress Notes:

_____

_____

_____

_____

_____

_____

_____

_____

_____

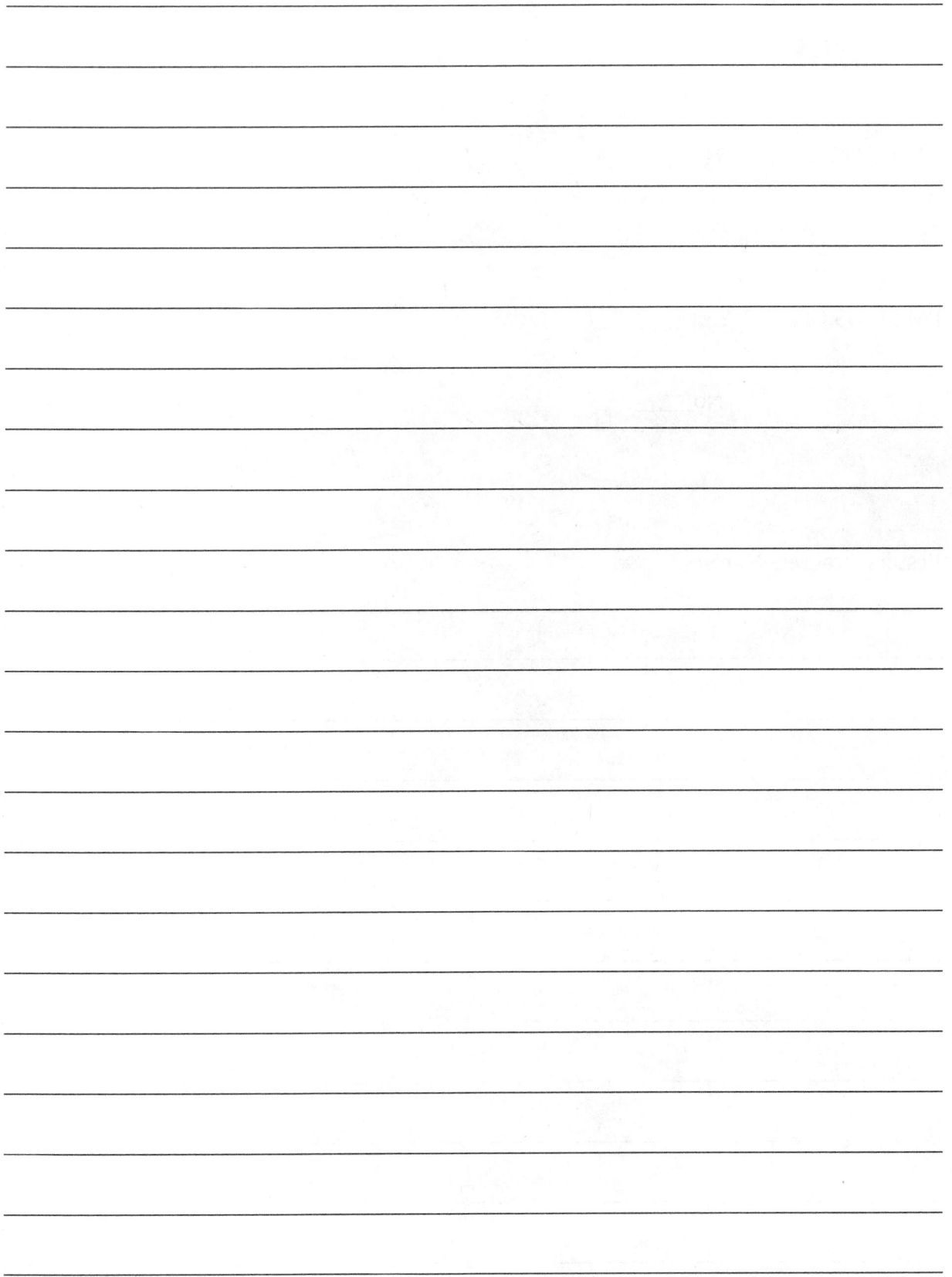

Date_____ Patient ID_____ Room Number_____

Medications   Administering   Mathematical

                Instructions   Computations

EST	Military	Notes	EST	Military	Notes	EST	Military	Notes	EST	Military	Notes
8:00 AM	08:00		3:15PM	15:15		10:15PM	22:15		5:15AM	05:15	
8:15 AM	08:15		3:30PM	15:30		10:30PM	22:30		5:30AM	05:30	
8:30AM	08:30		3:45PM	15:45		10:45PM	22:45		5:45AM	05:45	
8:45AM	08:45		4:00PM	16:00		11:00PM	23:00		6:00AM	06:00	
9:00AM	09:00		4:15PM	16:15		11:15PM	23:15		6:15AM	06:15	
9:15AM	09:15		4:30PM	16:30		11:30PM	23:30		6:30AM	06:30	
9:30AM	09:30		4:45PM	16:45		11:45PM	23:45		6:45AM	06:45	
9:45AM	09:45		5:00PM	17:00		12:00AM	24:00		7:00AM	07:00	
10:00AM	10:00		5:15PM	17:15		12:15AM	24:15		7:15AM	07:15	
10:15AM	10:15		5:30PM	17:30		12:30AM	24:30		730AM	07:30	
10:30AM	10:30		5:45PM	17:45		12:45AM	24:45		7:45AM	07:45	
10:45AM	10:45		6:00PM	18:00		1:00AM	01:00				
11:00AM	11:00		6:15PM	18:15		1:15AM	01:15				
11:15AM	11:15		6:30PM	18:30		1:30AM	01:30				
11:30AM	11:30		6:45PM	18:45		1:45AM	01:45				
11:45AM	11:45		7:00PM	19:00		2:00AM	02:00				
12:00PM	12:00		7:15PM	19:15		2:15AM	02:15				
12:15PM	12:15		7:30PM	19:30		2:45AM	02:45				
12:30PM	12:30		7:45PM	19:45		3:00AM	03:00				
12:45PM	12:45		8:00PM	20:00		3:15AM	03:15				
1:00PM	13:00		8:15PM	20:15		3:30AM	03:30				
1:15PM	13:15		8:30PM	20:30		3:45AM	03:45				
1:30PM	13:30		8:45PM	20:45		4:00AM	04:00				
1:45PM	13:45		9:00PM	21:00		4:15AM	04:15				
2:00PM	14:00		9:15PM	21:15		4:30AM	04:30				
2:15PM	14:15		9:30PM	21:30		4:45AM	04:45				
2:30PM	14:30		9:45PM	21:45		5:00AM	05:00				
2:45PM	14:45		10:00PM	22:00							
3:00PM	15:00										

Date_____   Patient ID_____   Room Number_____

AM MEDS GIVEN? Yes_____

                               No_____

PM MEDS GIVEN? Yes_____

                               No_____

Results/Progress Notes:

_____

_____

_____

_____

_____

_____

_____

_____

_____

_____

Date_____ Patient ID_____ Room Number_____

Medications	Administering Instructions	Mathematical Computations

EST	Military	Notes	EST	Military	Notes	EST	Military	Notes	EST	Military	Notes
8:00 AM	08:00		3:15PM	15:15		10:15PM	22:15		5:15AM	05:15	
8:15 AM	08:15		3:30PM	15:30		10:30PM	22:30		5:30AM	05:30	
8:30AM	08:30		3:45PM	15:45		10:45PM	22:45		5:45AM	05:45	
8:45AM	08:45		4:00PM	16:00		11:00PM	23:00		6:00AM	06:00	
9:00AM	09:00		4:15PM	16:15		11:15PM	23:15		6:15AM	06:15	
9:15AM	09:15		4:30PM	16:30		11:30PM	23:30		6:30AM	06:30	
9:30AM	09:30		4:45PM	16:45		11:45PM	23:45		6:45AM	06:45	
9:45AM	09:45		5:00PM	17:00		12:00AM	24:00		7:00AM	07:00	
10:00AM	10:00		5:15PM	17:15		12:15AM	24:15		7:15AM	07:15	
10:15AM	10:15		5:30PM	17:30		12:30AM	24:30		730AM	07:30	
10:30AM	10:30		5:45PM	17:45		12:45AM	24:45		7:45AM	07:45	
10:45AM	10:45		6:00PM	18:00		1:00AM	01:00				
11:00AM	11:00		6:15PM	18:15		1:15AM	01:15				
11:15AM	11:15		6:30PM	18:30		1:30AM	01:30				
11:30AM	11:30		6:45PM	18:45		1:45AM	01:45				
11:45AM	11:45		7:00PM	19:00		2:00AM	02:00				
12:00PM	12:00		7:15PM	19:15		2:15AM	02:15				
12:15PM	12:15		7:30PM	19:30		2:45AM	02:45				
12:30PM	12:30		7:45PM	19:45		3:00AM	03:00				
12:45PM	12:45		8:00PM	20:00		3:15AM	03:15				
1:00PM	13:00		8:15PM	20:15		3:30AM	03:30				
1:15PM	13:15		8:30PM	20:30		3:45AM	03:45				
1:30PM	13:30		8:45PM	20:45		4:00AM	04:00				
1:45PM	13:45		9:00PM	21:00		4:15AM	04:15				
2:00PM	14:00		9:15PM	21:15		4:30AM	04:30				
2:15PM	14:15		9:30PM	21:30		4:45AM	04:45				
2:30PM	14:30		9:45PM	21:45		5:00AM	05:00				
2:45PM	14:45		10:00PM	22:00							
3:00PM	15:00										

Date_____   Patient ID_____   Room Number_____

AM MEDS GIVEN? Yes_____

                  No_____

PM MEDS GIVEN? Yes_____

                  No_____

Results/Progress Notes:

_____

_____

_____

_____

_____

_____

_____

_____

_____

_____

Date_____ Patient ID_____ Room Number_____

Medications	Administering Instructions	Mathematical Computations

EST	Military	Notes	EST	Military	Notes	EST	Military	Notes	EST	Military	Notes
8:00 AM	08:00		3:15PM	15:15		10:15PM	22:15		5:15AM	05:15	
8:15 AM	08:15		3:30PM	15:30		10:30PM	22:30		5:30AM	05:30	
8:30AM	08:30		3:45PM	15:45		10:45PM	22:45		5:45AM	05:45	
8:45AM	08:45		4:00PM	16:00		11:00PM	23:00		6:00AM	06:00	
9:00AM	09:00		4:15PM	16:15		11:15PM	23:15		6:15AM	06:15	
9:15AM	09:15		4:30PM	16:30		11:30PM	23:30		6:30AM	06:30	
9:30AM	09:30		4:45PM	16:45		11:45PM	23:45		6:45AM	06:45	
9:45AM	09:45		5:00PM	17:00		12:00AM	24:00		7:00AM	07:00	
10:00AM	10:00		5:15PM	17:15		12:15AM	24:15		7:15AM	07:15	
10:15AM	10:15		5:30PM	17:30		12:30AM	24:30		730AM	07:30	
10:30AM	10:30		5:45PM	17:45		12:45AM	24:45		7:45AM	07:45	
10:45AM	10:45		6:00PM	18:00		1:00AM	01:00				
11:00AM	11:00		6:15PM	18:15		1:15AM	01:15				
11:15AM	11:15		6:30PM	18:30		1:30AM	01:30				
11:30AM	11:30		6:45PM	18:45		1:45AM	01:45				
11:45AM	11:45		7:00PM	19:00		2:00AM	02:00				
12:00PM	12:00		7:15PM	19:15		2:15AM	02:15				
12:15PM	12:15		7:30PM	19:30		2:45AM	02:45				
12:30PM	12:30		7:45PM	19:45		3:00AM	03:00				
12:45PM	12:45		8:00PM	20:00		3:15AM	03:15				
1:00PM	13:00		8:15PM	20:15		3:30AM	03:30				
1:15PM	13:15		8:30PM	20:30		3:45AM	03:45				
1:30PM	13:30		8:45PM	20:45		4:00AM	04:00				
1:45PM	13:45		9:00PM	21:00		4:15AM	04:15				
2:00PM	14:00		9:15PM	21:15		4:30AM	04:30				
2:15PM	14:15		9:30PM	21:30		4:45AM	04:45				
2:30PM	14:30		9:45PM	21:45		5:00AM	05:00				
2:45PM	14:45		10:00PM	22:00							
3:00PM	15:00										

Date_____ Patient ID_____ Room Number_____

AM MEDS GIVEN? Yes_____

                  No_____

PM MEDS GIVEN? Yes_____

                  No_____

Results/Progress Notes:

_____

_____

_____

_____

_____

_____

_____

_____

_____

_____

Date_____ Patient ID_____ Room Number_____

Medications   Administering   Mathematical

                     Instructions   Computations

EST	Military	Notes	EST	Military	Notes	EST	Military	Notes	EST	Military	Notes
8:00 AM	08:00		3:15PM	15:15		10:15PM	22:15		5:15AM	05:15	
8:15 AM	08:15		3:30PM	15:30		10:30PM	22:30		5:30AM	05:30	
8:30AM	08:30		3:45PM	15:45		10:45PM	22:45		5:45AM	05:45	
8:45AM	08:45		4:00PM	16:00		11:00PM	23:00		6:00AM	06:00	
9:00AM	09:00		4:15PM	16:15		11:15PM	23:15		6:15AM	06:15	
9:15AM	09:15		4:30PM	16:30		11:30PM	23:30		6:30AM	06:30	
9:30AM	09:30		4:45PM	16:45		11:45PM	23:45		6:45AM	06:45	
9:45AM	09:45		5:00PM	17:00		12:00AM	24:00		7:00AM	07:00	
10:00AM	10:00		5:15PM	17:15		12:15AM	24:15		7:15AM	07:15	
10:15AM	10:15		5:30PM	17:30		12:30AM	24:30		730AM	07:30	
10:30AM	10:30		5:45PM	17:45		12:45AM	24:45		7:45AM	07:45	
10:45AM	10:45		6:00PM	18:00		1:00AM	01:00				
11:00AM	11:00		6:15PM	18:15		1:15AM	01:15				
11:15AM	11:15		6:30PM	18:30		1:30AM	01:30				
11:30AM	11:30		6:45PM	18:45		1:45AM	01:45				
11:45AM	11:45		7:00PM	19:00		2:00AM	02:00				
12:00PM	12:00		7:15PM	19:15		2:15AM	02:15				
12:15PM	12:15		7:30PM	19:30		2:45AM	02:45				
12:30PM	12:30		7:45PM	19:45		3:00AM	03:00				
12:45PM	12:45		8:00PM	20:00		3:15AM	03:15				
1:00PM	13:00		8:15PM	20:15		3:30AM	03:30				
1:15PM	13:15		8:30PM	20:30		3:45AM	03:45				
1:30PM	13:30		8:45PM	20:45		4:00AM	04:00				
1:45PM	13:45		9:00PM	21:00		4:15AM	04:15				
2:00PM	14:00		9:15PM	21:15		4:30AM	04:30				
2:15PM	14:15		9:30PM	21:30		4:45AM	04:45				
2:30PM	14:30		9:45PM	21:45		5:00AM	05:00				
2:45PM	14:45		10:00PM	22:00							
3:00PM	15:00										

Date_____ Patient ID_____ Room Number_____

AM MEDS GIVEN? Yes_____

               No_____

PM MEDS GIVEN? Yes_____

               No_____

Results/Progress Notes:

_____

_____

_____

_____

_____

_____

_____

_____

_____

_____

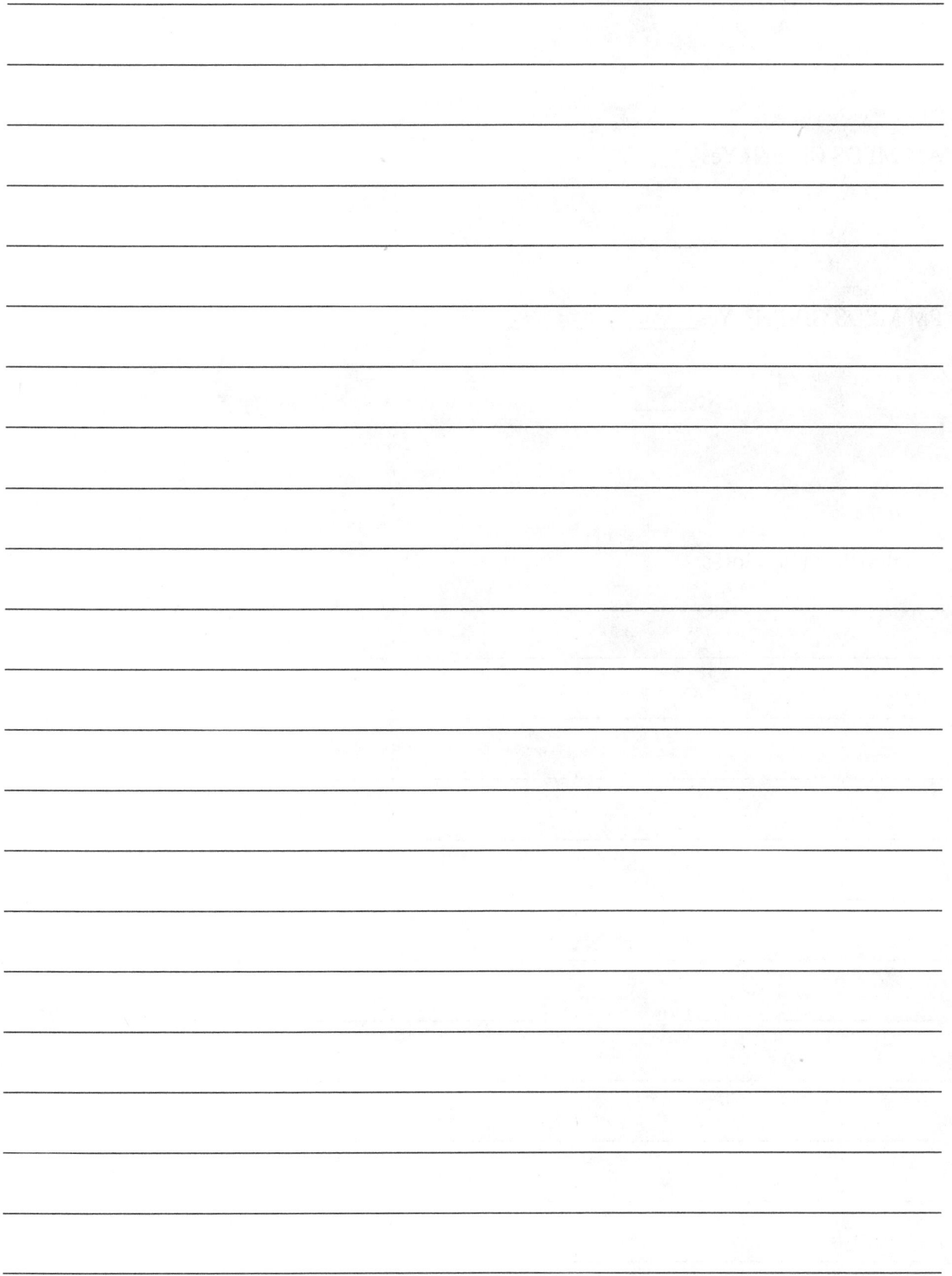

Date_____ Patient ID_____ Room Number_____

Medications	Administering Instructions

Mathematical Computations

EST	Military	Notes	EST	Military	Notes	EST	Military	Notes	EST	Military	Notes
8:00 AM	08:00		3:15PM	15:15		10:15PM	22:15		5:15AM	05:15	
8:15 AM	08:15		3:30PM	15:30		10:30PM	22:30		5:30AM	05:30	
8:30AM	08:30		3:45PM	15:45		10:45PM	22:45		5:45AM	05:45	
8:45AM	08:45		4:00PM	16:00		11:00PM	23:00		6:00AM	06:00	
9:00AM	09:00		4:15PM	16:15		11:15PM	23:15		6:15AM	06:15	
9:15AM	09:15		4:30PM	16:30		11:30PM	23:30		6:30AM	06:30	
9:30AM	09:30		4:45PM	16:45		11:45PM	23:45		6:45AM	06:45	
9:45AM	09:45		5:00PM	17:00		12:00AM	24:00		7:00AM	07:00	
10:00AM	10:00		5:15PM	17:15		12:15AM	24:15		7:15AM	07:15	
10:15AM	10:15		5:30PM	17:30		12:30AM	24:30		730AM	07:30	
10:30AM	10:30		5:45PM	17:45		12:45AM	24:45		7:45AM	07:45	
10:45AM	10:45		6:00PM	18:00		1:00AM	01:00				
11:00AM	11:00		6:15PM	18:15		1:15AM	01:15				
11:15AM	11:15		6:30PM	18:30		1:30AM	01:30				
11:30AM	11:30		6:45PM	18:45		1:45AM	01:45				
11:45AM	11:45		7:00PM	19:00		2:00AM	02:00				
12:00PM	12:00		7:15PM	19:15		2:15AM	02:15				
12:15PM	12:15		7:30PM	19:30		2:45AM	02:45				
12:30PM	12:30		7:45PM	19:45		3:00AM	03:00				
12:45PM	12:45		8:00PM	20:00		3:15AM	03:15				
1:00PM	13:00		8:15PM	20:15		3:30AM	03:30				
1:15PM	13:15		8:30PM	20:30		3:45AM	03:45				
1:30PM	13:30		8:45PM	20:45		4:00AM	04:00				
1:45PM	13:45		9:00PM	21:00		4:15AM	04:15				
2:00PM	14:00		9:15PM	21:15		4:30AM	04:30				
2:15PM	14:15		9:30PM	21:30		4:45AM	04:45				
2:30PM	14:30		9:45PM	21:45		5:00AM	05:00				
2:45PM	14:45		10:00PM	22:00							
3:00PM	15:00										

Date_____ Patient ID_____ Room Number_____

AM MEDS GIVEN? Yes_____

No_____

PM MEDS GIVEN? Yes_____

No_____

Results/Progress Notes:

_____

_____

_____

_____

_____

_____

_____

_____

_____

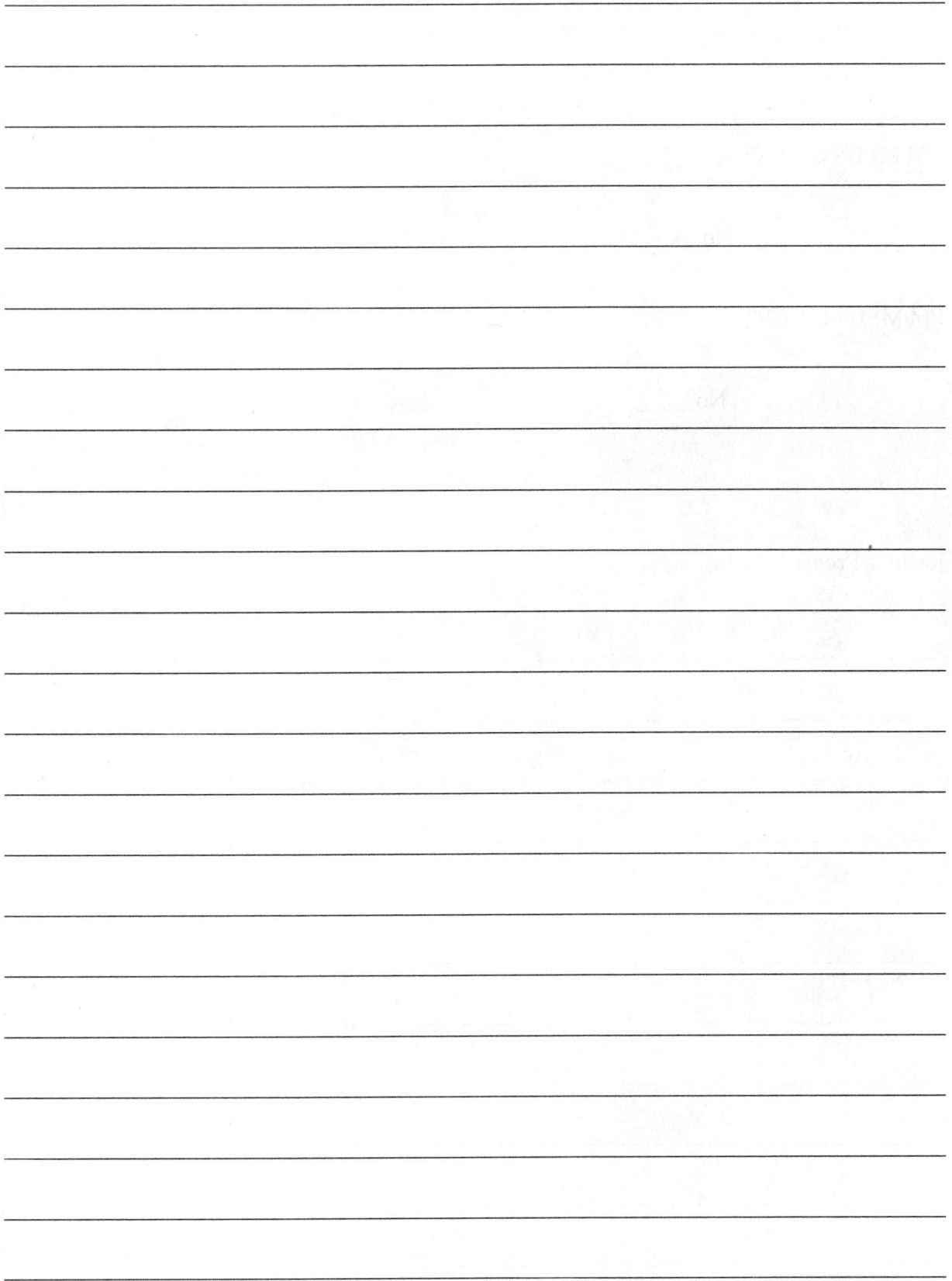

Date_____ Patient ID_____ Room Number_____

Medications	Administering Instructions	Mathematical Computations

EST	Military	Notes	EST	Military	Notes	EST	Military	Notes	EST	Military	Notes
8:00 AM	08:00		3:15PM	15:15		10:15PM	22:15		5:15AM	05:15	
8:15 AM	08:15		3:30PM	15:30		10:30PM	22:30		5:30AM	05:30	
8:30AM	08:30		3:45PM	15:45		10:45PM	22:45		5:45AM	05:45	
8:45AM	08:45		4:00PM	16:00		11:00PM	23:00		6:00AM	06:00	
9:00AM	09:00		4:15PM	16:15		11:15PM	23:15		6:15AM	06:15	
9:15AM	09:15		4:30PM	16:30		11:30PM	23:30		6:30AM	06:30	
9:30AM	09:30		4:45PM	16:45		11:45PM	23:45		6:45AM	06:45	
9:45AM	09:45		5:00PM	17:00		12:00AM	24:00		7:00AM	07:00	
10:00AM	10:00		5:15PM	17:15		12:15AM	24:15		7:15AM	07:15	
10:15AM	10:15		5:30PM	17:30		12:30AM	24:30		730AM	07:30	
10:30AM	10:30		5:45PM	17:45		12:45AM	24:45		7:45AM	07:45	
10:45AM	10:45		6:00PM	18:00		1:00AM	01:00				
11:00AM	11:00		6:15PM	18:15		1:15AM	01:15				
11:15AM	11:15		6:30PM	18:30		1:30AM	01:30				
11:30AM	11:30		6:45PM	18:45		1:45AM	01:45				
11:45AM	11:45		7:00PM	19:00		2:00AM	02:00				
12:00PM	12:00		7:15PM	19:15		2:15AM	02:15				
12:15PM	12:15		7:30PM	19:30		2:45AM	02:45				
12:30PM	12:30		7:45PM	19:45		3:00AM	03:00				
12:45PM	12:45		8:00PM	20:00		3:15AM	03:15				
1:00PM	13:00		8:15PM	20:15		3:30AM	03:30				
1:15PM	13:15		8:30PM	20:30		3:45AM	03:45				
1:30PM	13:30		8:45PM	20:45		4:00AM	04:00				
1:45PM	13:45		9:00PM	21:00		4:15AM	04:15				
2:00PM	14:00		9:15PM	21:15		4:30AM	04:30				
2:15PM	14:15		9:30PM	21:30		4:45AM	04:45				
2:30PM	14:30		9:45PM	21:45		5:00AM	05:00				
2:45PM	14:45		10:00PM	22:00							
3:00PM	15:00										

Date_____ Patient ID_____ Room Number_____

AM MEDS GIVEN? Yes_____

No_____

PM MEDS GIVEN? Yes_____

No_____

Results/Progress Notes:

_____

_____

_____

_____

_____

_____

_____

_____

_____

_____

Date_____ Patient ID_____ Room Number_____

Medications	Administering Instructions

Mathematical Computations

EST	Military	Notes	EST	Military	Notes	EST	Military	Notes	EST	Military	Notes
8:00 AM	08:00		3:15PM	15:15		10:15PM	22:15		5:15AM	05:15	
8:15 AM	08:15		3:30PM	15:30		10:30PM	22:30		5:30AM	05:30	
8:30AM	08:30		3:45PM	15:45		10:45PM	22:45		5:45AM	05:45	
8:45AM	08:45		4:00PM	16:00		11:00PM	23:00		6:00AM	06:00	
9:00AM	09:00		4:15PM	16:15		11:15PM	23:15		6:15AM	06:15	
9:15AM	09:15		4:30PM	16:30		11:30PM	23:30		6:30AM	06:30	
9:30AM	09:30		4:45PM	16:45		11:45PM	23:45		6:45AM	06:45	
9:45AM	09:45		5:00PM	17:00		12:00AM	24:00		7:00AM	07:00	
10:00AM	10:00		5:15PM	17:15		12:15AM	24:15		7:15AM	07:15	
10:15AM	10:15		5:30PM	17:30		12:30AM	24:30		730AM	07:30	
10:30AM	10:30		5:45PM	17:45		12:45AM	24:45		7:45AM	07:45	
10:45AM	10:45		6:00PM	18:00		1:00AM	01:00				
11:00AM	11:00		6:15PM	18:15		1:15AM	01:15				
11:15AM	11:15		6:30PM	18:30		1:30AM	01:30				
11:30AM	11:30		6:45PM	18:45		1:45AM	01:45				
11:45AM	11:45		7:00PM	19:00		2:00AM	02:00				
12:00PM	12:00		7:15PM	19:15		2:15AM	02:15				
12:15PM	12:15		7:30PM	19:30		2:45AM	02:45				
12:30PM	12:30		7:45PM	19:45		3:00AM	03:00				
12:45PM	12:45		8:00PM	20:00		3:15AM	03:15				
1:00PM	13:00		8:15PM	20:15		3:30AM	03:30				
1:15PM	13:15		8:30PM	20:30		3:45AM	03:45				
1:30PM	13:30		8:45PM	20:45		4:00AM	04:00				
1:45PM	13:45		9:00PM	21:00		4:15AM	04:15				
2:00PM	14:00		9:15PM	21:15		4:30AM	04:30				
2:15PM	14:15		9:30PM	21:30		4:45AM	04:45				
2:30PM	14:30		9:45PM	21:45		5:00AM	05:00				
2:45PM	14:45		10:00PM	22:00							
3:00PM	15:00										

Date_____   Patient ID_____   Room Number_____

AM MEDS GIVEN? Yes_____

                No_____

PM MEDS GIVEN? Yes_____

                No_____

Results/Progress Notes:

_____

_____

_____

_____

_____

_____

_____

_____

_____

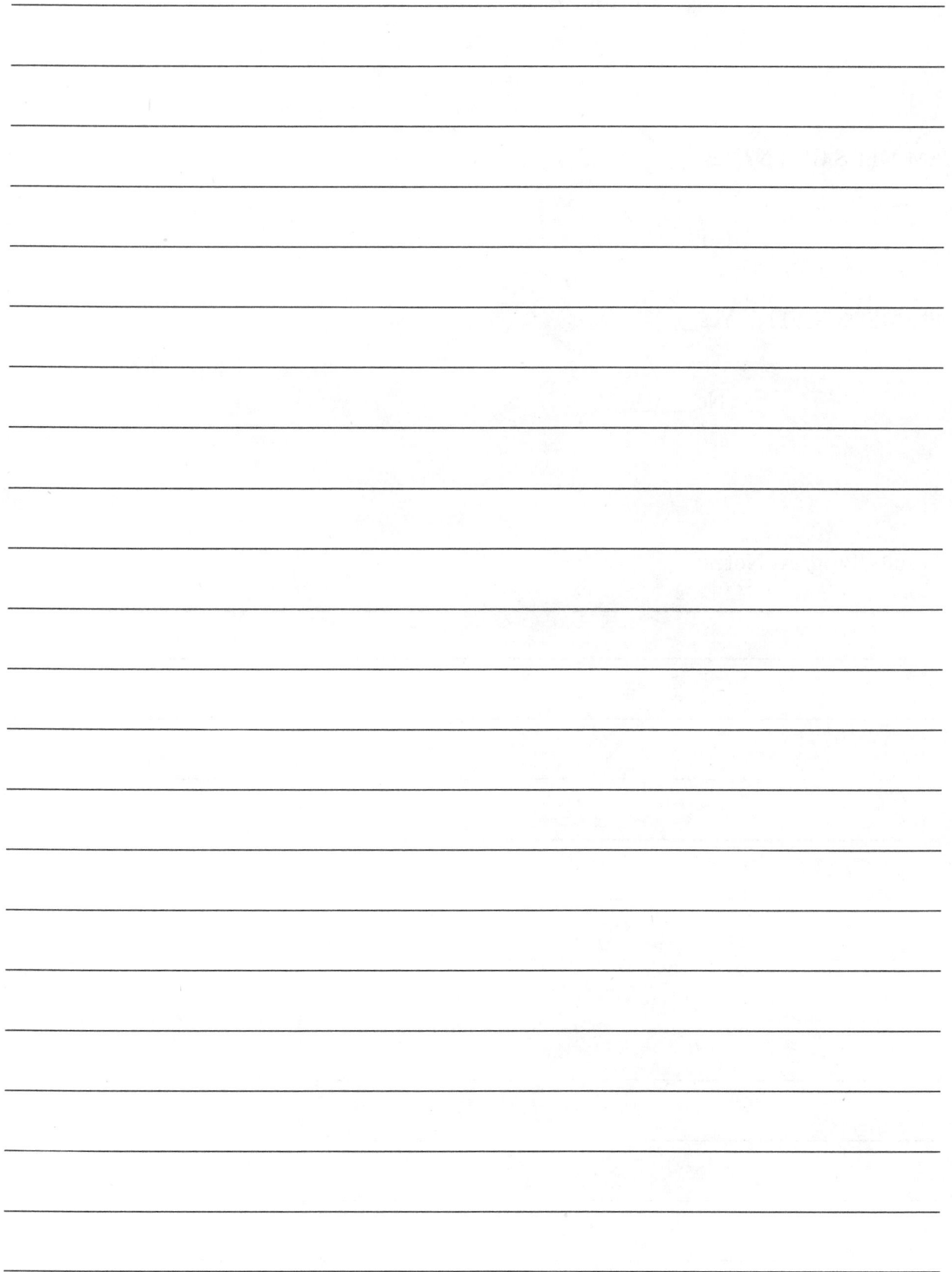

Date_____ Patient ID_____ Room Number_____

Medications	Administering Instructions	Mathematical Computations

EST	Military	Notes	EST	Military	Notes	EST	Military	Notes	EST	Military	Notes
8:00 AM	08:00		3:15PM	15:15		10:15PM	22:15		5:15AM	05:15	
8:15 AM	08:15		3:30PM	15:30		10:30PM	22:30		5:30AM	05:30	
8:30AM	08:30		3:45PM	15:45		10:45PM	22:45		5:45AM	05:45	
8:45AM	08:45		4:00PM	16:00		11:00PM	23:00		6:00AM	06:00	
9:00AM	09:00		4:15PM	16:15		11:15PM	23:15		6:15AM	06:15	
9:15AM	09:15		4:30PM	16:30		11:30PM	23:30		6:30AM	06:30	
9:30AM	09:30		4:45PM	16:45		11:45PM	23:45		6:45AM	06:45	
9:45AM	09:45		5:00PM	17:00		12:00AM	24:00		7:00AM	07:00	
10:00AM	10:00		5:15PM	17:15		12:15AM	24:15		7:15AM	07:15	
10:15AM	10:15		5:30PM	17:30		12:30AM	24:30		730AM	07:30	
10:30AM	10:30		5:45PM	17:45		12:45AM	24:45		7:45AM	07:45	
10:45AM	10:45		6:00PM	18:00		1:00AM	01:00				
11:00AM	11:00		6:15PM	18:15		1:15AM	01:15				
11:15AM	11:15		6:30PM	18:30		1:30AM	01:30				
11:30AM	11:30		6:45PM	18:45		1:45AM	01:45				
11:45AM	11:45		7:00PM	19:00		2:00AM	02:00				
12:00PM	12:00		7:15PM	19:15		2:15AM	02:15				
12:15PM	12:15		7:30PM	19:30		2:45AM	02:45				
12:30PM	12:30		7:45PM	19:45		3:00AM	03:00				
12:45PM	12:45		8:00PM	20:00		3:15AM	03:15				
1:00PM	13:00		8:15PM	20:15		3:30AM	03:30				
1:15PM	13:15		8:30PM	20:30		3:45AM	03:45				
1:30PM	13:30		8:45PM	20:45		4:00AM	04:00				
1:45PM	13:45		9:00PM	21:00		4:15AM	04:15				
2:00PM	14:00		9:15PM	21:15		4:30AM	04:30				
2:15PM	14:15		9:30PM	21:30		4:45AM	04:45				
2:30PM	14:30		9:45PM	21:45		5:00AM	05:00				
2:45PM	14:45		10:00PM	22:00							
3:00PM	15:00										

Date_____ Patient ID_____ Room Number_____

AM MEDS GIVEN? Yes_____

No_____

PM MEDS GIVEN? Yes_____

No_____

Results/Progress Notes:

_____

_____

_____

_____

_____

_____

_____

_____

_____

_____

Date_____ Patient ID_____ Room Number_____

Medications	Administering Instructions	Mathematical Computations

EST	Military	Notes	EST	Military	Notes	EST	Military	Notes	EST	Military	Notes
8:00 AM	08:00		3:15PM	15:15		10:15PM	22:15		5:15AM	05:15	
8:15 AM	08:15		3:30PM	15:30		10:30PM	22:30		5:30AM	05:30	
8:30AM	08:30		3:45PM	15:45		10:45PM	22:45		5:45AM	05:45	
8:45AM	08:45		4:00PM	16:00		11:00PM	23:00		6:00AM	06:00	
9:00AM	09:00		4:15PM	16:15		11:15PM	23:15		6:15AM	06:15	
9:15AM	09:15		4:30PM	16:30		11:30PM	23:30		6:30AM	06:30	
9:30AM	09:30		4:45PM	16:45		11:45PM	23:45		6:45AM	06:45	
9:45AM	09:45		5:00PM	17:00		12:00AM	24:00		7:00AM	07:00	
10:00AM	10:00		5:15PM	17:15		12:15AM	24:15		7:15AM	07:15	
10:15AM	10:15		5:30PM	17:30		12:30AM	24:30		730AM	07:30	
10:30AM	10:30		5:45PM	17:45		12:45AM	24:45		7:45AM	07:45	
10:45AM	10:45		6:00PM	18:00		1:00AM	01:00				
11:00AM	11:00		6:15PM	18:15		1:15AM	01:15				
11:15AM	11:15		6:30PM	18:30		1:30AM	01:30				
11:30AM	11:30		6:45PM	18:45		1:45AM	01:45				
11:45AM	11:45		7:00PM	19:00		2:00AM	02:00				
12:00PM	12:00		7:15PM	19:15		2:15AM	02:15				
12:15PM	12:15		7:30PM	19:30		2:45AM	02:45				
12:30PM	12:30		7:45PM	19:45		3:00AM	03:00				
12:45PM	12:45		8:00PM	20:00		3:15AM	03:15				
1:00PM	13:00		8:15PM	20:15		3:30AM	03:30				
1:15PM	13:15		8:30PM	20:30		3:45AM	03:45				
1:30PM	13:30		8:45PM	20:45		4:00AM	04:00				
1:45PM	13:45		9:00PM	21:00		4:15AM	04:15				
2:00PM	14:00		9:15PM	21:15		4:30AM	04:30				
2:15PM	14:15		9:30PM	21:30		4:45AM	04:45				
2:30PM	14:30		9:45PM	21:45		5:00AM	05:00				
2:45PM	14:45		10:00PM	22:00							
3:00PM	15:00										

Date_____ Patient ID_____ Room Number_____

AM MEDS GIVEN? Yes_____

No_____

PM MEDS GIVEN? Yes_____

No_____

Results/Progress Notes:

_____

_____

_____

_____

_____

_____

_____

_____

_____

Date_____ Patient ID_____ Room Number_____

Medications	Administering Instructions	Mathematical Computations

EST	Military	Notes	EST	Military	Notes	EST	Military	Notes	EST	Military	Notes
8:00 AM	08:00		3:15PM	15:15		10:15PM	22:15		5:15AM	05:15	
8:15 AM	08:15		3:30PM	15:30		10:30PM	22:30		5:30AM	05:30	
8:30AM	08:30		3:45PM	15:45		10:45PM	22:45		5:45AM	05:45	
8:45AM	08:45		4:00PM	16:00		11:00PM	23:00		6:00AM	06:00	
9:00AM	09:00		4:15PM	16:15		11:15PM	23:15		6:15AM	06:15	
9:15AM	09:15		4:30PM	16:30		11:30PM	23:30		6:30AM	06:30	
9:30AM	09:30		4:45PM	16:45		11:45PM	23:45		6:45AM	06:45	
9:45AM	09:45		5:00PM	17:00		12:00AM	24:00		7:00AM	07:00	
10:00AM	10:00		5:15PM	17:15		12:15AM	24:15		7:15AM	07:15	
10:15AM	10:15		5:30PM	17:30		12:30AM	24:30		730AM	07:30	
10:30AM	10:30		5:45PM	17:45		12:45AM	24:45		7:45AM	07:45	
10:45AM	10:45		6:00PM	18:00		1:00AM	01:00				
11:00AM	11:00		6:15PM	18:15		1:15AM	01:15				
11:15AM	11:15		6:30PM	18:30		1:30AM	01:30				
11:30AM	11:30		6:45PM	18:45		1:45AM	01:45				
11:45AM	11:45		7:00PM	19:00		2:00AM	02:00				
12:00PM	12:00		7:15PM	19:15		2:15AM	02:15				
12:15PM	12:15		7:30PM	19:30		2:45AM	02:45				
12:30PM	12:30		7:45PM	19:45		3:00AM	03:00				
12:45PM	12:45		8:00PM	20:00		3:15AM	03:15				
1:00PM	13:00		8:15PM	20:15		3:30AM	03:30				
1:15PM	13:15		8:30PM	20:30		3:45AM	03:45				
1:30PM	13:30		8:45PM	20:45		4:00AM	04:00				
1:45PM	13:45		9:00PM	21:00		4:15AM	04:15				
2:00PM	14:00		9:15PM	21:15		4:30AM	04:30				
2:15PM	14:15		9:30PM	21:30		4:45AM	04:45				
2:30PM	14:30		9:45PM	21:45		5:00AM	05:00				
2:45PM	14:45		10:00PM	22:00							
3:00PM	15:00										

Date_____ Patient ID_____ Room Number_____

AM MEDS GIVEN? Yes_____

              No_____

PM MEDS GIVEN? Yes_____

              No_____

Results/Progress Notes:

_____

_____

_____

_____

_____

_____

_____

_____

_____

_____

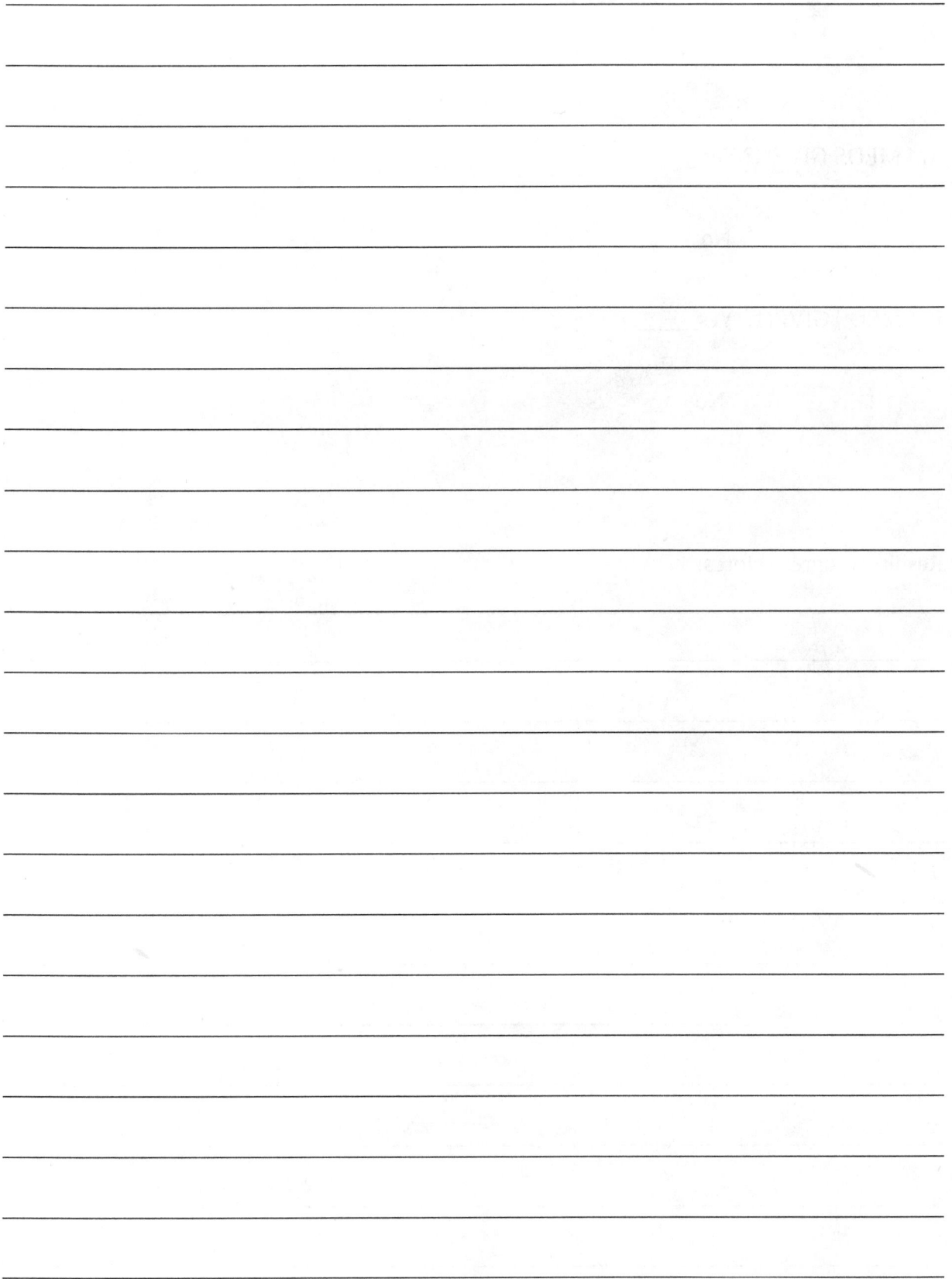

Date_____   Patient ID_____   Room Number_____

Medications   Administering   Mathematical

Instructions   Computations

EST	Military	Notes	EST	Military	Notes	EST	Military	Notes	EST	Military	Notes
8:00 AM	08:00		3:15PM	15:15		10:15PM	22:15		5:15AM	05:15	
8:15 AM	08:15		3:30PM	15:30		10:30PM	22:30		5:30AM	05:30	
8:30AM	08:30		3:45PM	15:45		10:45PM	22:45		5:45AM	05:45	
8:45AM	08:45		4:00PM	16:00		11:00PM	23:00		6:00AM	06:00	
9:00AM	09:00		4:15PM	16:15		11:15PM	23:15		6:15AM	06:15	
9:15AM	09:15		4:30PM	16:30		11:30PM	23:30		6:30AM	06:30	
9:30AM	09:30		4:45PM	16:45		11:45PM	23:45		6:45AM	06:45	
9:45AM	09:45		5:00PM	17:00		12:00AM	24:00		7:00AM	07:00	
10:00AM	10:00		5:15PM	17:15		12:15AM	24:15		7:15AM	07:15	
10:15AM	10:15		5:30PM	17:30		12:30AM	24:30		730AM	07:30	
10:30AM	10:30		5:45PM	17:45		12:45AM	24:45		7:45AM	07:45	
10:45AM	10:45		6:00PM	18:00		1:00AM	01:00				
11:00AM	11:00		6:15PM	18:15		1:15AM	01:15				
11:15AM	11:15		6:30PM	18:30		1:30AM	01:30				
11:30AM	11:30		6:45PM	18:45		1:45AM	01:45				
11:45AM	11:45		7:00PM	19:00		2:00AM	02:00				
12:00PM	12:00		7:15PM	19:15		2:15AM	02:15				
12:15PM	12:15		7:30PM	19:30		2:45AM	02:45				
12:30PM	12:30		7:45PM	19:45		3:00AM	03:00				
12:45PM	12:45		8:00PM	20:00		3:15AM	03:15				
1:00PM	13:00		8:15PM	20:15		3:30AM	03:30				
1:15PM	13:15		8:30PM	20:30		3:45AM	03:45				
1:30PM	13:30		8:45PM	20:45		4:00AM	04:00				
1:45PM	13:45		9:00PM	21:00		4:15AM	04:15				
2:00PM	14:00		9:15PM	21:15		4:30AM	04:30				
2:15PM	14:15		9:30PM	21:30		4:45AM	04:45				
2:30PM	14:30		9:45PM	21:45		5:00AM	05:00				
2:45PM	14:45		10:00PM	22:00							
3:00PM	15:00										

Date_____ Patient ID_____ Room Number_____

AM MEDS GIVEN? Yes_____

No_____

PM MEDS GIVEN? Yes_____

No_____

Results/Progress Notes:

_____

_____

_____

_____

_____

_____

_____

_____

_____

_____

Date_____ Patient ID_____ Room Number_____

Medications	Administering Instructions	Mathematical Computations

EST	Military	Notes	EST	Military	Notes	EST	Military	Notes	EST	Military	Notes
8:00 AM	08:00		3:15PM	15:15		10:15PM	22:15		5:15AM	05:15	
8:15 AM	08:15		3:30PM	15:30		10:30PM	22:30		5:30AM	05:30	
8:30AM	08:30		3:45PM	15:45		10:45PM	22:45		5:45AM	05:45	
8:45AM	08:45		4:00PM	16:00		11:00PM	23:00		6:00AM	06:00	
9:00AM	09:00		4:15PM	16:15		11:15PM	23:15		6:15AM	06:15	
9:15AM	09:15		4:30PM	16:30		11:30PM	23:30		6:30AM	06:30	
9:30AM	09:30		4:45PM	16:45		11:45PM	23:45		6:45AM	06:45	
9:45AM	09:45		5:00PM	17:00		12:00AM	24:00		7:00AM	07:00	
10:00AM	10:00		5:15PM	17:15		12:15AM	24:15		7:15AM	07:15	
10:15AM	10:15		5:30PM	17:30		12:30AM	24:30		730AM	07:30	
10:30AM	10:30		5:45PM	17:45		12:45AM	24:45		7:45AM	07:45	
10:45AM	10:45		6:00PM	18:00		1:00AM	01:00				
11:00AM	11:00		6:15PM	18:15		1:15AM	01:15				
11:15AM	11:15		6:30PM	18:30		1:30AM	01:30				
11:30AM	11:30		6:45PM	18:45		1:45AM	01:45				
11:45AM	11:45		7:00PM	19:00		2:00AM	02:00				
12:00PM	12:00		7:15PM	19:15		2:15AM	02:15				
12:15PM	12:15		7:30PM	19:30		2:45AM	02:45				
12:30PM	12:30		7:45PM	19:45		3:00AM	03:00				
12:45PM	12:45		8:00PM	20:00		3:15AM	03:15				
1:00PM	13:00		8:15PM	20:15		3:30AM	03:30				
1:15PM	13:15		8:30PM	20:30		3:45AM	03:45				
1:30PM	13:30		8:45PM	20:45		4:00AM	04:00				
1:45PM	13:45		9:00PM	21:00		4:15AM	04:15				
2:00PM	14:00		9:15PM	21:15		4:30AM	04:30				
2:15PM	14:15		9:30PM	21:30		4:45AM	04:45				
2:30PM	14:30		9:45PM	21:45		5:00AM	05:00				
2:45PM	14:45		10:00PM	22:00							
3:00PM	15:00										

Date_____   Patient ID_____   Room Number_____

AM MEDS GIVEN? Yes_____

                         No_____

PM MEDS GIVEN? Yes_____

                      No_____

Results/Progress Notes:

_____

_____

_____

_____

_____

_____

_____

_____

_____

_____

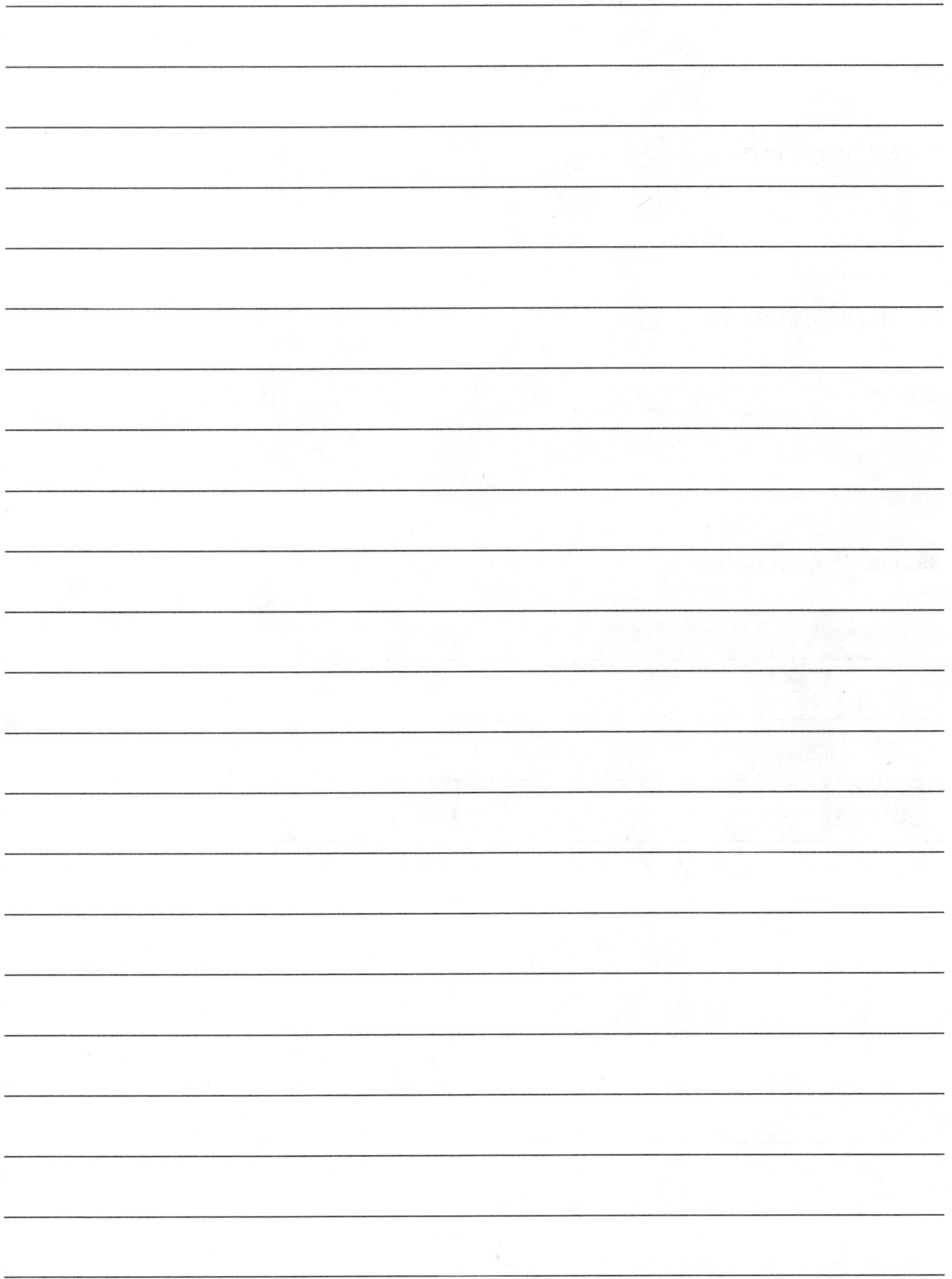

Date_____   Patient ID_____   Room Number_____

Medications	Administering Instructions	Mathematical Computations

EST	Military	Notes	EST	Military	Notes	EST	Military	Notes	EST	Military	Notes
8:00 AM	08:00		3:15PM	15:15		10:15PM	22:15		5:15AM	05:15	
8:15 AM	08:15		3:30PM	15:30		10:30PM	22:30		5:30AM	05:30	
8:30AM	08:30		3:45PM	15:45		10:45PM	22:45		5:45AM	05:45	
8:45AM	08:45		4:00PM	16:00		11:00PM	23:00		6:00AM	06:00	
9:00AM	09:00		4:15PM	16:15		11:15PM	23:15		6:15AM	06:15	
9:15AM	09:15		4:30PM	16:30		11:30PM	23:30		6:30AM	06:30	
9:30AM	09:30		4:45PM	16:45		11:45PM	23:45		6:45AM	06:45	
9:45AM	09:45		5:00PM	17:00		12:00AM	24:00		7:00AM	07:00	
10:00AM	10:00		5:15PM	17:15		12:15AM	24:15		7:15AM	07:15	
10:15AM	10:15		5:30PM	17:30		12:30AM	24:30		730AM	07:30	
10:30AM	10:30		5:45PM	17:45		12:45AM	24:45		7:45AM	07:45	
10:45AM	10:45		6:00PM	18:00		1:00AM	01:00				
11:00AM	11:00		6:15PM	18:15		1:15AM	01:15				
11:15AM	11:15		6:30PM	18:30		1:30AM	01:30				
11:30AM	11:30		6:45PM	18:45		1:45AM	01:45				
11:45AM	11:45		7:00PM	19:00		2:00AM	02:00				
12:00PM	12:00		7:15PM	19:15		2:15AM	02:15				
12:15PM	12:15		7:30PM	19:30		2:45AM	02:45				
12:30PM	12:30		7:45PM	19:45		3:00AM	03:00				
12:45PM	12:45		8:00PM	20:00		3:15AM	03:15				
1:00PM	13:00		8:15PM	20:15		3:30AM	03:30				
1:15PM	13:15		8:30PM	20:30		3:45AM	03:45				
1:30PM	13:30		8:45PM	20:45		4:00AM	04:00				
1:45PM	13:45		9:00PM	21:00		4:15AM	04:15				
2:00PM	14:00		9:15PM	21:15		4:30AM	04:30				
2:15PM	14:15		9:30PM	21:30		4:45AM	04:45				
2:30PM	14:30		9:45PM	21:45		5:00AM	05:00				
2:45PM	14:45		10:00PM	22:00							
3:00PM	15:00										

Date_____   Patient ID_____   Room Number_____

AM MEDS GIVEN? Yes_____

               No_____

PM MEDS GIVEN? Yes_____

               No_____

Results/Progress Notes:

_____

_____

_____

_____

_____

_____

_____

_____

_____

_____

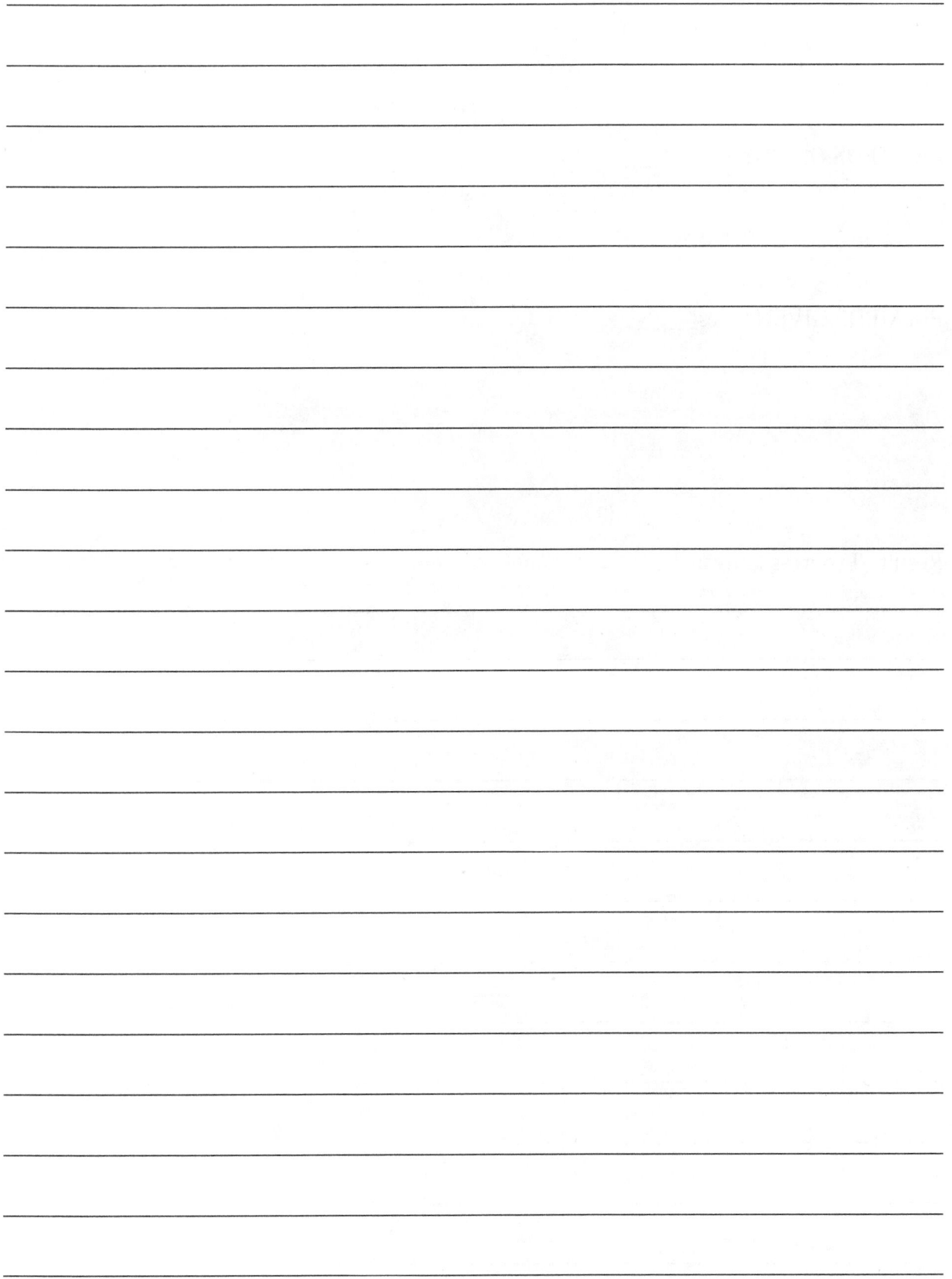

Date_____ Patient ID_____ Room Number_____

Medications   Administering   Mathematical

Instructions   Computations

EST	Military	Notes	EST	Military	Notes	EST	Military	Notes	EST	Military	Notes
8:00 AM	08:00		3:15PM	15:15		10:15PM	22:15		5:15AM	05:15	
8:15 AM	08:15		3:30PM	15:30		10:30PM	22:30		5:30AM	05:30	
8:30AM	08:30		3:45PM	15:45		10:45PM	22:45		5:45AM	05:45	
8:45AM	08:45		4:00PM	16:00		11:00PM	23:00		6:00AM	06:00	
9:00AM	09:00		4:15PM	16:15		11:15PM	23:15		6:15AM	06:15	
9:15AM	09:15		4:30PM	16:30		11:30PM	23:30		6:30AM	06:30	
9:30AM	09:30		4:45PM	16:45		11:45PM	23:45		6:45AM	06:45	
9:45AM	09:45		5:00PM	17:00		12:00AM	24:00		7:00AM	07:00	
10:00AM	10:00		5:15PM	17:15		12:15AM	24:15		7:15AM	07:15	
10:15AM	10:15		5:30PM	17:30		12:30AM	24:30		730AM	07:30	
10:30AM	10:30		5:45PM	17:45		12:45AM	24:45		7:45AM	07:45	
10:45AM	10:45		6:00PM	18:00		1:00AM	01:00				
11:00AM	11:00		6:15PM	18:15		1:15AM	01:15				
11:15AM	11:15		6:30PM	18:30		1:30AM	01:30				
11:30AM	11:30		6:45PM	18:45		1:45AM	01:45				
11:45AM	11:45		7:00PM	19:00		2:00AM	02:00				
12:00PM	12:00		7:15PM	19:15		2:15AM	02:15				
12:15PM	12:15		7:30PM	19:30		2:45AM	02:45				
12:30PM	12:30		7:45PM	19:45		3:00AM	03:00				
12:45PM	12:45		8:00PM	20:00		3:15AM	03:15				
1:00PM	13:00		8:15PM	20:15		3:30AM	03:30				
1:15PM	13:15		8:30PM	20:30		3:45AM	03:45				
1:30PM	13:30		8:45PM	20:45		4:00AM	04:00				
1:45PM	13:45		9:00PM	21:00		4:15AM	04:15				
2:00PM	14:00		9:15PM	21:15		4:30AM	04:30				
2:15PM	14:15		9:30PM	21:30		4:45AM	04:45				
2:30PM	14:30		9:45PM	21:45		5:00AM	05:00				
2:45PM	14:45		10:00PM	22:00							
3:00PM	15:00										

Date_____ Patient ID_____ Room Number_____

AM MEDS GIVEN? Yes_____

No_____

PM MEDS GIVEN? Yes_____

No_____

Results/Progress Notes:

_____

_____

_____

_____

_____

_____

_____

_____

_____

www.ingramcontent.com/pod-product-compliance
Lightning Source LLC
Chambersburg PA
CBHW080242270326
41926CB00020B/4336